Postpartum Nursing
Health Care of Women

Joellen Beck Watson Hawkins, R.N.C., Ph.D., F.A.A.N., is a professor in the graduate program, School of Nursing, Boston College, specializing in women's health care. She obtained a master's degree in maternal-child health nursing, and a Ph.D., from Boston College, and has taught and worked at Boston Lying-In Hospital. Dr. Hawkins was active in the 1960s and '70s childbirth education movement, and for the past several years has maintained an active practice as a Certified Ob/Gyn Nurse Practitioner. In addition, she has served on the faculties of Salve Regina College and the University of Connecticut. She has written or collaborated on a dozen books, including *Maternity and Gynecological Nursing, Health Care of Women: Labor and Delivery,* and *Clinical Experiences in Collegiate Nursing Education.*

Beverly Gorvine, R.N., M.S., is currently the Associate Administrator for Nursing Services for the Cambridge Hospital, Cambridge, Massachusetts. She received a master's degree in maternal-child health nursing from Boston College, has taught and worked at Boston Lying-In Hospital, and has served as a labor coach in practice with a physician. Ms. Gorvine has taught at Boston College, and served as Clinical Director of Maternal-Child Health at Mt. Auburn Hospital and St. Elizabeth's Hospital (Cambridge and Brighton, Massachusetts). She has been a member of a team for the Regional Project to Improve the Quality of Maternal Child Health Care, funded by the U.S. Public Health Service, and is the co-author of *Maternal-Newborn Nursing: PreTest Self-Assessment and Review,* and *Health Care of Women: Labor and Delivery.*

Carolyn Currier-Dagrosa, R.N., M.S., teaches at Marymount College of Virginia. She has a master's degree in maternal-child health from Boston University, and is presently a doctoral candidate in the School of Education at the University of Connecticut. She contributed to *Current Practice in Pediatric Nursing.*

Patricia Fleming, R.N., M.S., is Clinical Services Manager for Visiting Nurse Association, Inc., Providence, Rhode Island. The recipient of an M.S. from the University of Connecticut in maternal-child health nursing, she has been a head nurse on a postpartum newborn unit.

Rachel F. Schiffman, R.N., M.S., is a faculty member at Rhode Island College in the Department of Nursing. She holds a master's degree in maternal-child health nursing from the University of Connecticut where she is currently a doctoral student. Previously a staff nurse and inservice coordinator at Women and Infants Hospital of Rhode Island, she practiced with emphasis on postpartum, newborn, and antenatal care.

Postpartum Nursing
Health Care of Women

Joellen W. Hawkins, R.N.C., Ph.D., F.A.A.N.
Beverly Gorvine, R.N., M.S.
with
Carolyn Currier-Dagrosa, R.N., M.S.
Patricia Fleming, R.N., M.S.
Rachel F. Schiffman, R.N., M.S.

Springer Publishing Company
New York

Springer Publishing Company, Inc.
200 Park Avenue South
New York, New York 10003

85 86 87 88 89 / 10 9 8 7 6 5 4 3 2 1

Library of Congress Cataloging in Publication Data

Hawkins, Joellen Watson.
Postpartum nursing.
Includes bibliographies and index.
1. Postnatal care. 2. Obstetrical nursing. 3. Puerperium. I. Gorvine, Beverly F. II. Title. [DNLM: 1. Obstetrical Nursing. 2. Postnatal Care. 3. Puerperium. WY 157.3 H393p]
RG801.H38 1985 610.73'678 84-14038
ISBN 0-8261-4690-2 (pbk.)

Printed in the United States of America

Photo Credits

Bruce L. and Lynne Beck, Marie and James R. Knight, Janet and Douglas Beck, Karen and Richard Ramos, Louise and Eddy Baduski

To our families
for continued patience, care, and support.

Contents

Preface

This book is designed as a guide for clinical practice in the postpartum area based on a nursing model. It is written for nurses working or preparing to work in the postpartum setting, for graduate students focusing on childbearing families, and for undergraduate students electing an advanced clinical component in the maternity setting.

The object of the book is to explore theory in the field, describe application of one nursing model to a practice setting, and delineate nursing interventions for families in the postpartum setting. This book is planned to supplement and complement basic texts covering postpartum nursing. As such, it explores in depth the time of the puerperium through the steps of nursing process. It is our hope that it will be a useful guide for clinical practice in the challenging and exciting postpartum setting.

Acknowledgments

To our students and colleagues whose input has been invaluable to the development of this book, we say thank you.

We are especially indebted to Janice Bittner, our typist, who supports us through project after project with her tremendous patience and skill.

To Carole Saltz, formerly of Springer Publishing Company, we owe our gratitude for her belief in us, her helpful comments and suggestions, and her support.

Most of all, to friends and families, as always, we owe our deepest gratitude for their continuing love and support through all our projects.

Joellen W. Hawkins

Beverly Gorvine

1

The Puerperium as a Time of Crisis

Introduction

The puerperium is a time of reflection, of reliving the pregnancy and birth experiences, a time of adjustment to new roles, and accommodation of the family to a new member. It represents a developmental milestone for the man and woman, something of an end to childhood and a symbolic, as well as actual, taking on of one of the many possible roles and responsibilities society ascribes to adults, that of parenting. Grandparents and other members of the extended family are acquiring new roles as well. A firstborn child now has a sibling. Blended families increase the complexity of role designation; the new baby may be a step sib or a half brother or sister. Parents may now be adjusting to having "our" child as well as his and/or hers.

Nurses who are providers of care for families in this transitional and disruptive period have unique skills and expertise to offer. The preparation and support families receive during the puerperium is important in augmenting the coping strategies they have used in previous times of change. Furthermore, assessment of adaptations of the woman, her infant, and the family will be important to planning for utilization of resources after discharge should the continued potential for crisis seem evident. An optimal experience during the hospitalized portion of the puerperium is one that prepares the family for growth through the developmental stages that acquisition of a new family member represents.

A Historical Overview of Postpartum Care

In the nineteenth century, hospitals attracted only a small percentage of women. Their image was tarnished by the dangers of puerperal fever and a reputation for giving refuge to homeless women (Wertz & Wertz, 1979, pp. 132–133). Fewer than 5 percent of women delivered in hospitals; today the figures are more than reversed.

The popularity of hospitals for the birthing event is complex. Hospitals for some offered a cleaner, safer environment for delivery and recuperation. With the advent of the use of general anesthesia in the last century and the use of medications and regional anesthetics during this century, hospital care gained in popularity. In hospital, women were promised painless childbirth and the marvels of twilight sleep. Clinical advances in use of forceps, surgical and medical asepsis, and cesarean section all but mandated the hospital setting for their utilization or implementation. In 1920 Dr. Joseph De Lee urged routine use of forceps and episiotomy (Wertz & Wertz, 1979, p. 141).

Convenience for physicians specializing in obstetrical practices became an issue. X-ray equipment, transfusion, anesthesia, and drugs became tools of the trade; their place, in the hospital (Wertz & Wertz, 1979, p. 144).

Scarcity of and decline in the use of household help, the emerging middle-class housewife who did her own housework, and the opening up of more types of employment for women made the hospital an attractive alternative to home delivery. There the woman would be cared for during the two weeks or longer lying-in period. It was a time to recuperate while others performed the chores. Amenities such as bedside telephones, hospital beds, porches, and nursing care lured women to the hospital to deliver painlessly and be cared for for several weeks. Poor women, faced with declining services by midwives, chose hospital delivery as the only alternative. These women sometimes suffered at the hands of inexperienced house staff and a lack of standards for care (Wertz & Wertz, 1979, pp. 156–173).

The rise in the popularity and necessity of hospital deliveries was paralleled by the evolution of the profession of nursing. Beginning in 1874 the Boston Training School for Nurses provided to Boston Lying-in Hospital a pupil every two months. By 1885, the hospital had established its own school under the direction of a Miss Emily A. Rogers, graduate of Boston City (Irving, 1942, p. 191). De Lee's *Obstetrics for Nurses*, first published in 1904, included an extensive section on the puerperium and care of the woman and her infant. In the fourth edition, published in 1916, the timing of ambulation is discussed. It is stated that most women are allowed up at the tenth day, but other accoucheurs allow it only in the third or fourth week (De Lee, 1916, p. 148).

Fullerton's book on obstetric nursing was already in its sixth edition by 1904. Management of the lying-in is discussed in detail, including rest, visitors, involution, the lochia, micturition, constipation, nipple and breast care, afterpains, bedsores, puerperal mania, puerperal fever, ulcers, and milk leg (pp. 146–179). Duration of lying-in was to be six weeks of which at least two would be in bed (p. 150).

In 1917, the National League of Nursing Education was recommending inclusion of obstetric nursing as a required component of its *Curriculum Guide for Schools of Nursing.* Early in the history of education for professional nursing, therefore, obstetric nursing was considered an important component in the preparation for practice.

Use of a Nursing Model

The practice of nursing should extend beyond successful completion of tasks. Likewise, if we are to practice *nursing* rather than limiting our interventions to those that are physician designated or prescribed, we need to be able to articulate what it is that we offer to clients that is unique and even superior to services of other health care providers. Utilization of a conceptual model for practice gives structure to what we do, helps generate research questions that arise from concerns or problems we experience in developing and implementing nursing strategies, and provides a sound basis in theory.

The medical model is illness oriented, focuses on diagnosis and treatment of disease, and has curing as its main interactional component. Nursing should be wellness and health oriented, focus on assessment and interventions, and include components of caring, comforting, teaching, counseling, and coordinating (Mauksch, 1977). Thus, nursing models incorporate these components and focus on nursing assessment, interventions, and evaluation of care. A nursing model includes four essential components—the individual, health, environment, and nursing—and defines each of these within the context of the development of the particular model. Several nursing models have been developed. Roy, Orem, Rogers, Neuman, and Kinlein are some of the names associated with the development of nursing theory and models for practice. References on nursing models are included in the bibliography.

Conceptual models for nursing are based on theories drawn from a number of disciplines. The building of a theoretical basis for practice within the context of a model is similar to the process of synthesis in education, requiring that students draw on material from courses in social and physical sciences, humanities, and the arts as well as from nursing courses in carrying out steps of nursing process in order to provide nursing care for clients. Theories are selected for the strengths and dimensions they bring to the art and science of professional nursing practice.

Crisis Nursing Model

The crisis nursing model has been chosen for the framework of this book on nursing care during the peurperium for several reasons. Utilization of a nursing model for practice accentuates the strengths and unique skills and knowledge nurses bring to their professional practice with clients. Use of a model provides a framework for practice and guides the development of forms for record keeping such as Kardex cards, teaching modules, care plans, and anecdotal notes. A sound theoretical basis for practice helps nurses to share with clients, peers, and other providers what they as nurses do for clients that is unique and superior to services offered by other health care providers and how nursing care complements those services.

The crisis model is particularly appropriate for nursing practice with childbearing and childrearing individuals and families because it is a developmental model. Theories incorporated in the model include: developmental task, crisis, role, biological and social systems, body image, psychoanalytic elements, stress, and rites of passage (Koehne & Fawcett, 1972). All of these theories have important applications for individuals and families in the childbearing and childrearing years. Both authors have had experience with implementation of this model in practice settings. Much has been written about the crisis potential for individuals and families in the decision-making and implementation phases of parenting. Baird (1976) writes of the potential for crisis in the childrearing cycle and offers crisis intervention theory as an appropriate basis for interventions with individuals and families. The crisis model serves as a useful example of incorporation of a nursing model in practice because it is a logical model, based on theories that are a part of the educational and practice backgrounds of most if not all professional nurses.

Finally, the crisis model has applications not only for clients, but also for nurses themselves. The new graduate may find herself in a crisis state when confronted with the discrepancy between her practice skills and the role requirements thrust upon her. Staff members may need to have their coping mechanisms augmented in order to remain in precrisis when tragedies occur in the maternity unit, ordinarily a relatively happy place.

Components of the model. The four necessary components for a nursing model to exist are defined as they are utilized in the crisis model in Table 1.1. The stages of crisis as they may be viewed for clients during the puerperium across the wellness–illness–wellness continuum are represented in Figure 1.1. It is important in using the model to elicit or assess not only the woman's perceptions of the events of pregnancy, labor and birth, and the puerperium but also those of other family members as they deal with changing roles, and the infant's responses to birth and extrauterine life. The Brazelton Neonatal Assessment Scale is one useful tool in assessing the infant's responses to (perceptions of) his or her environment (1973).

The goal of nursing intervention utilizing this model is maintenance of all members of the family in precrisis or, if crisis occurs, mobilizing resources to lead to resolution of crisis, growth, and health. Nursing focuses on augmenting self-sufficiency, rather than intervening when it is appropriate for clients to participate in or be responsible for their own care. This would include fostering the comfort of parent(s) in the care of their infant prior to discharge. Virginia Henderson conceptualizes the client as a health care agent and nursing as "Complementing the patient by supplying what he [she] needs" (1966, p. 21).

Table 1.2 gives some examples of common hazardous events that affect childbearing/childrearing individuals and families during the puerperium. Of course, attention must also be given to other situational hazardous events such as a death in the family, loss of a job, moving to a new location, and so on which will affect the individual or family responses to the developmental tasks imposed by a birth. The Holmes and Rahe Scale which rates such hazardous events is included in Appendix C. Any individual with over 200 points is at greater risk for crisis including biophysical crisis such as illness. In a study of life changes associated with pregnancy, Williams and colleagues (1975) utilized a sample of women during the postpartum period, half of whom had delivered at term and half prematurely. The two groups reported similar magnitudes of life change occurring during their pregnancies and for the two years preceding conception. Interestingly, those women who had experienced medical problems during pregnancy did report significantly higher life change during pregnancy and one year prior to conception than did those women who experienced no medical problems (p. 129). In a similar study, Nuckolls, Cassel, and Kaplan found that women with high life change scores and low psychosocial asset scores were

Table 1.1 Essential Components of a Nursing Model: Crisis

Individual (Man)	Environment	Health	Nursing
physiological	internal and external forces	exists in relation to illness and environment	process based on sciences and humanities
psychological	alters, altered by individual	illness = prolonged state of disequilibrium or maladaptation	augments coping behaviors
social being		individual's perceptions affect definition of health	mobilizes resources
open system within environment		maintenance of equilibrium and successful coping indices of health	intervenes to provide for needs to prevent crisis, restore wellness
holistic		wellness-illness-wellness model	intervenes in crisis to restore maximum possible level of wellness post-crisis
dynamic			process interactional
active role			manipulate external or internal environment to help achieve or maintain higher level of wellness, prevent crisis
exists on developmental continuum which is orderly and consistent			independent and interdependent functions
participant--uses problem-solving and decision-making			

more likely to experience complications during pregnancy than those women with high psychosocial asset scores (1972). Hazardous events may also be characterized as risk factors with the potential for crisis, whether biophysical or psychosocial. Nursing is directed toward augmenting coping mechanisms or providing interventions to maintain a precrisis state.

Factors that affect the potential for an optimal level of wellness for individuals and families in the puerperium appear in Table 1.3. This list is not all inclusive, as it would be different for each individual and each family. Part of the health assessment process includes eliciting information about support systems and resources. Other members of the health team can assist the family in mobilizing resources such as money to pay the hospital bills. Referral to the visiting nurse service is useful for home follow-up. Day care will allow the woman to return to work or relieve her of the care of several small children.

Sometimes it is helpful to use a schematic drawing to represent the components of an interactional system such as a postpartum unit. Figure 1.2 is such a drawing. The nurse(s), woman, her infant, and family and significant others are the primary figures who interact in a typical postpartum unit. Other health care providers interact, but usually in a more peripheral way unless crisis threatens or occurs and additional resources must be mobilized. These other providers may be inside or outside of the hospital setting and the postpartum unit. Usually they are not an integral part of the unit, so they are represented by a circle surrounding the inner circles of the unit. The circles are like semipermeable membranes permitting flow in and out. Family and significant others may spend a great deal of time on the unit, particularly the father of the child, so they are considered (or should be) an integral part of the unit even though their contact is more limited than that of the woman, her infant, and nurses. For the duration of the hospital stay, only the woman and her infant are on the unit 24 hours a day (usually), as nursing shifts change. Such a drawing helps to visualize the interchange between each of the components and to include it in the assessment process when relevant. The drawing for a family when the infant requires transfer to a neonatal intensive care unit (NICU) would be dramatically different and helps to point out the potential for crisis for the woman and her family (Figure 1.3).

In practice, such models are useful to lend perspective to the potential forces women and their families may be subjected to and to understand the plethora of interactions forced upon families and the importance of communication at other levels to maximize health and promote the highest level of wellness.

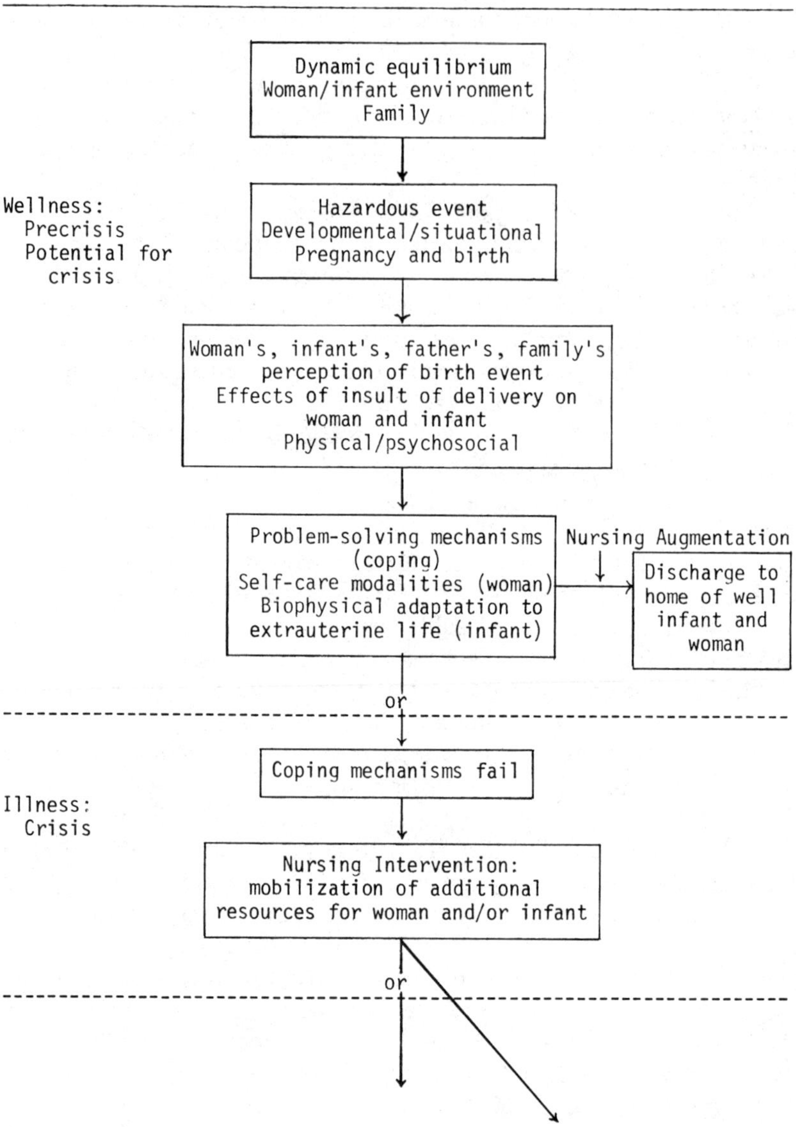

Figure 1.1 Use of crisis theory in a wellness–illness–wellness continuum for postpartum care.

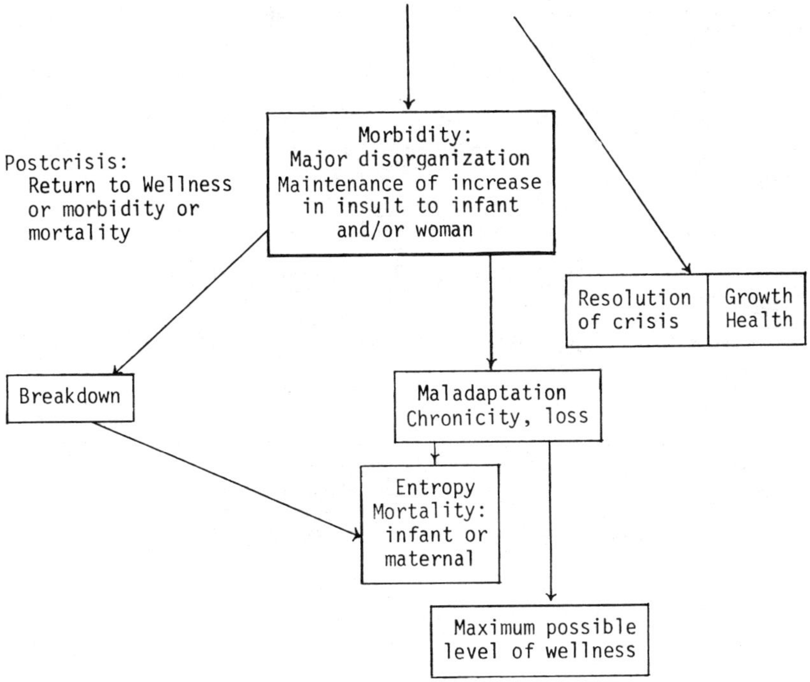

*Adapted from the Crisis Model, The University of Connecticut School of Nursing.

Figure 1.1 (Continued)

Table 1.2 Examples of Hazardous Events Affecting Individuals and Families During the Puerperium

Developmental	Situational
sexual activity	infection
intimacy	toxemia
assumption of parenting roles and responsiblities	respiratory distress syndrome
adaptation to extrauterine life	prematurity
role change and adaptation	coagulation defects/venous disorders
attachment of parents and infant	genetic aberrations
trust vs. mistrust	congenital anomalies
generativity vs. stagnation	Caesarean section
alterations in body image	psychosis
	sterilization
	stillbirth

The Puerperium and Its Potential for Crisis

Assumption of the parenting role is part of the developmental task Erikson calls generativity versus stagnation (1963, p. 267). The production of a child may follow close upon or be simultaneous with the evolution of a sense of identity—one of the tasks ascribed to adolescence—and intimacy—which overlaps adolescence and young adulthood (Erikson, 1963, pp. 261, 263). The potential for crisis is greater when the woman and her partner are absorbed in the tasks of identity and intimacy and have thrust upon them responsibility for the next generation. Risks for the teenaged parent are greater from a psychosocial as well as a biophysical perspective. Teens are pushed out of childhood and into adulthood when pregnancy occurs. Birth and puerperium end the childhood of new parents.

Support systems present in cultures preserving the integrity of extended families are generally not available to women bearing children in our society. The potential for crisis is heightened in the absence of support and adequate role modeling of parenting skills. Mercer (1981) discusses the tasks of the postpartum period for the woman. These include grief work as the result of parting with her fantasies about her infant and her postpartum body; her infant's performance; her mothering skills; a redefining of roles; and resumption of responsibilities upon discharge from the hospital. Each of these tasks has the potential for crisis and each has implications for nursing interventions.

Reorganization of the family social system is inevitable when a new baby is born. Roles are reassigned, new roles as parents taken on, priorities shift, needs are met in alternate ways, values may have to be realigned, and status changes occur (Clark, 1971, p. 45). The pregnant woman, once the center of attention, is no longer pregnant and the focus shifts to the new infant. The woman may have to curtail her career, at least temporarily, or make child care arrangements and let go of some of the tasks of mothering. The man may take on new responsibilities within the household. Priorities must shift to accommo-

Table 1.3 Factors That Affect Potential for Optimal Level of Wellness During the Puerperium

Intrinsic	Extrinsic
genetics	socio-economic status
nutrition	resources
	financial
sex	social
	religious
race	political
	cultural
weight	
	education
gestational age	
	peers
	family/significant others
	environment
	home
	work
	hospital
	school
	health care system
	geographic
	neighborhood

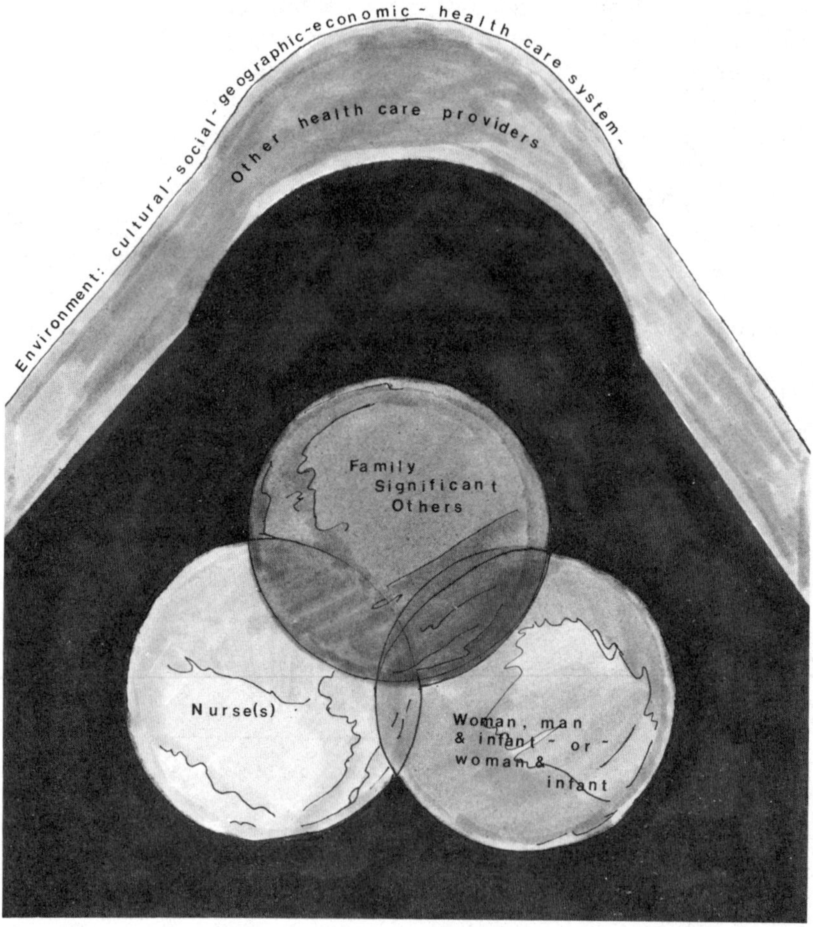

Figure 1.2 Nursing care for women, their infants, and families during the puerperium. (Marcy-Leigh Rolling, artist. Copyright retained by artist.)

date the responsibilities parenthood entails. All of these consequences carry with them the potential for crisis. Additionally, as Clark points out, reorganization is dynamic (p. 45). The disruption of the dyad or other composition of the family social system is, however, necessary in order to incorporate the new family member. If it does not occur as in failure or inadequacy of parent–child attachment, or if it is disrupted by prolonged hospitalization of either child or mother, the potential for crisis is even greater.

Coupled with reorganization of the household is reorganization of the woman's identity from woman, wife, worker, perhaps professional, to woman, wife, worker, professional, *and* mother (Ludington-Hoe, 1977, p. 1171). Similar reorganization occurs for the man, but it is usual that women assume more of the responsibilities of household and child care at present in our society, so the effects on his role functioning may not be as profound. More men are assuming responsibility for child care or sharing it equally with their partners, however, so the potential for role conflict and crisis for these men will be greater than for those for

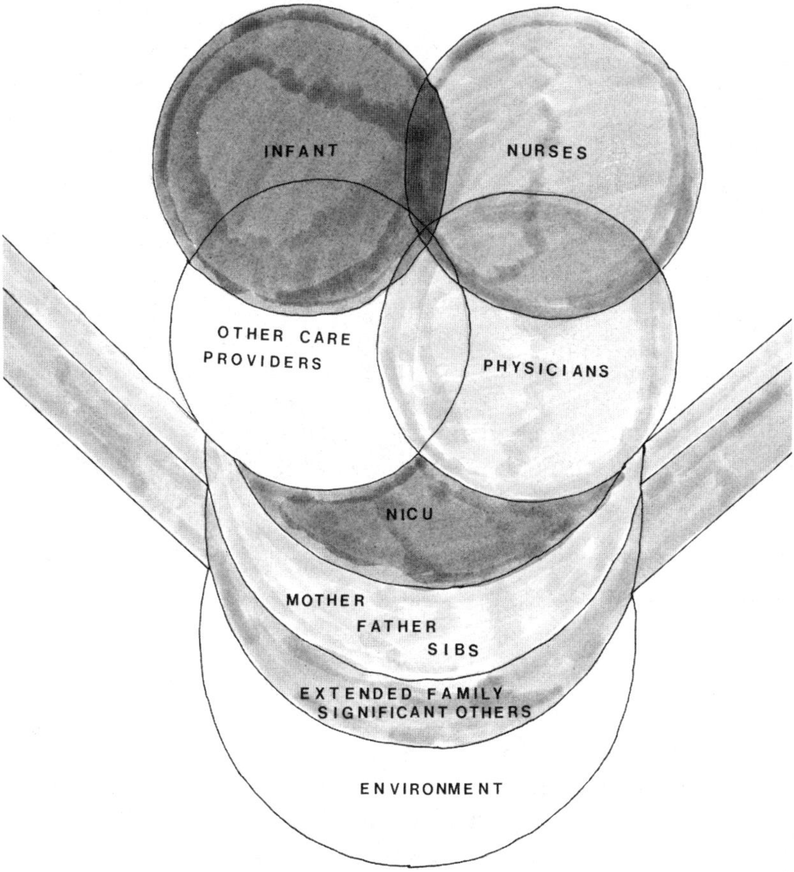

Figure 1.3 Infant in a neonatal intensive care unit. (Marcy-Leigh Rolling, artist. Copyright retained by artist.)

whom fathering is little more than a biological fact and/or financial responsibility.

The woman's figure postpartum "may cause her more anguish than her pregnant figure did" (Bishop, 1976, p. 1785). Fawcett's findings suggest that women underestimate the actual amount of space their bodies occupy early in the puerperium (1978, p. 232). This may be a reflection of dissatisfaction with body image or a discrepancy between real and imagined ideal. The anticipation that prepregnant contours will be assumed shortly after delivery gives way to reality and the potential for crisis surrounding body image.

Another source of potential crisis is disruption/resumption of expressions of intimacy for the couple through genital intercourse. Some couples may have had to abstain prior to delivery due to pregnancy complications or discomfort and fear. Resumption of intercourse is dependent upon the couple's psychological readiness as well as the woman's biophysical well-being. Issues of sexuality and contraception should be addressed during the puerperium. The couple need to be prepared for the physiological changes, both temporary and permanent, which affect sexual function and response (Inglis, 1980, pp. 298–299).

The potential for biophysical crisis for both the woman and her infant exists during the puerperium. The leading causes of maternal morbidity and mortality are still infection, hemorrhage, and toxemia. Risks to the woman are increased when there is superimposed on pregnancy a preexisting situational hazardous event such as diabetes, hypertension, or cardiac disease. The infant's potential for crisis is increased when premature delivery occurs or when the infant is small for gestational age or has suffered a biophysical insult, hereditary or acquired. Examples include Down's syndrome, respiratory distress syndrome, and periods of hypoxia or anoxia. The potential for crisis may be predictable when a pregnancy or fetus is designated as at-risk or unpredictable, as in the occurrence of a knot in the cord or laceration of the cervix.

Summary

There is evidence in the research literature that parents as well as health care providers view the birth of a child as a maturational crisis or at least an event with the potential for crisis (Dyer, 1965, p. 323; LeMasters, 1965, pp. 111–117). A complexity of tasks is required to complete the period of role transition during the puerperium. This complexity of tasks adds to the already tremendous potential for crisis involved in the birth of an infant (Rhode & Groenjes-Finke, 1980, p. 23). The developmental events are compounded by potential or actual superimposed situational events such as premature birth, hemorrhage, infection, birth injury, or anomaly. Nurses can significantly affect the outcomes by augmenting coping mechanisms to maintain the family resources and intervening when crisis occurs, and by promoting resolution and growth or at least an optimal level of wellness postcrisis.

References

Baird, S. F. Emotional crisis and maternal-child nursing. *Journal of Obstetric, Gynecologic and Neonatal Nursing*, 1976, *5*(1), 30–39.

Bishop, B. A guide to assessing parenting capabilities. *American Journal of Nursing*, 1976, *76*(11), 1784–1787.

Brazelton, T. B. *Neonatal behavioral assessment scale*. London: William Heinemann, Ltd., 1973.

Clark, A. L. Stresses and conflicts: Their relevance to the expanding family. In A. L. Clark (Ed.), *Maturational crisis of childbearing*. Honolulu: University of Hawaii, 1971, pp. 45–57.

Committee on Curriculum of the National League of Nursing Education. *A curriculum guide for schools of nursing*. New York: National League of Nursing Education, 1917.

De Lee, J. B. *Obstetrics for nurses* (4th ed.). Philadelphia: W. B. Saunders, 1916.

Dyer, E. D. Parenthood as crisis: A re-study. In H. J. Parad (Ed.), *Crisis intervention: Selected readings*. New York: Family Service Association of America, 1965, pp. 312–323.

Erikson, E. H. *Childhood and society* (2nd ed.). New York: W. W. Norton, 1963.

Fawcett, J. Body image and the pregnant couple. *The American Journal of Maternal Child Nursing*, 1978, *3*(4), 227–233.

Fullerton, A. M. *A handbook of obstetric nursing for nurses, students and mothers* (6th ed.). Philadelphia: P. Blakeston's Sons & Co., 1904.

Henderson, V. *The nature of nursing*. New York: Macmillan, 1966.

Inglis, T. Post partum sexuality. *Journal of Obstetric, Gynecologic and Neonatal Nursing*, 1980, *9*(5), 298–300.

Irving, F. C. *Safe deliverance*. Boston: Houghton Mifflin, 1942.

Koehne, N., & Fawcett, J. *Discussion of crisis theory* (mimeographed). Storrs: University of Connecticut School of Nursing, 1972.

LeMasters, E. E. Parenthood as crisis. In H. J. Parad (Ed.), *Crisis intervention: Selected readings*. New York: Family Service Association of America, 1965, pp. 111–117.

Ludington-Hoe, S. M. Postpartum: Development of maternicity. *American Journal of Nursing*, 1977, *77*(7), 1171–1174.

Mauksch, I. *Unpublished speech given to Alpha Chi Chapter, Sigma Theta Tau*, 28 February 1977, Boston College.

Mercer, R. T. The nurse and maternal tasks of early postpartum. *The American*

Journal of Maternal Child Nursing, 1981, *6*(5), 341–345.

Nuckolls, K. B., Cassel, J., & Kaplan, B. H. Psychosocial assets, life crisis and the prognosis of pregnancy. *American Journal of Epidemiology*, 1972, *95*(5), 431–441.

Rhode, M. A., & Groenjes-Finke, J. M. Evaluation of nurse-initiated telephone calls to postpartum women. *Issues in Health Care of Women*, 1980, *2*(2), 23–41.

Wertz, R. W., & Wertz, D. C. *Lying-in: A history of childbirth in America*. New York: Schocken, 1979.

Williams, C. C., Williams, R. A., Griswold, M. J., & Holmes, T. H. Pregnancy and life change. *Journal of Psychosomatic Research*, 1975, *19*(2), 123–129.

2

The Puerperium and Neonatal Periods: Biophysical Aspects

Introduction

Birth is a beginning, for the baby in his or her transition into extrauterine life and for the woman in her biophysical adaptation to a nonpregnant state and in her role. Just as the infant can never return to a fetal state, so the woman will never again be a nullipara. The biophysical changes which occur are closely interwoven with the psychosocial/cultural aspects. In this chapter, the biophysical adaptations that both woman and infant must successfully accomplish to remain in a precrisis state will be explored in order to provide a foundation for all that is to follow in discussions of developmental tasks and hazardous events.

Adaptation of the Woman's Body to a Nonpregnant State

Profound changes occur very precipitously in the moments following completion of the third stage of labor. The woman's body, divested of the placenta, membranes, and dependent fetus must make rapid adaptations if hemorrhage is to be avoided. Adjustment of cardiovascular, respiratory, endocrine, musculoskeletal, gastrointestinal, and neurological systems to providing for the needs of or accommodating to only one individual must occur. The potential for crisis is significant. Prompt assessments and appropriate augmentation and/or interventions are part of the nursing care that is directed toward support of an optimal level of functioning during the biophysical transitions. Knowledge of the transitional processes provides a basis for nursing care and is essential for the first step of assessment to occur.

Uterus

Emptied of its contents, this highly vascular organ which has so recently held the products of conception is highly vulnerable as a site for hemorrhage and infection. With the birth of the placenta, the major source of progesterones and estrogens is removed. Responding to this hormonal shift, the anterior pituitary releases prolactin or lactogenic hormone. This activity is, in part, coupled with psychoneural mechanisms which the baby's sucking initiates (Netter, 1965, p. 121).

The level of oxytocins present in plasma can be demonstrated to be 165 units per milliliter at 40 weeks of gestation (Kumaresan et al., 1974, pp. 215–223). Sucking stimulates the pituitary to release oxytocin, which causes the myometrium to contract. Oxytocin is produced in the hypothalamus and stored and released from the posterior pituitary (Danforth & Hendricks, 1977, p. 533). In some way not yet completely understood, oxytocin activates the contractile system of the myometrium. The placenta appears to have oxytocin-destroying capacities through enzymes it produces. It can be hypothesized, therefore, that with the delivery of the placenta, oxytocin released from the posterior pituitary and present in the woman's plasma will act on the myometrium to cause it to contract. Administration of exogenous oxytocin during the puerperium does cause uterine contraction and is one treatment in the presence of an atonic uterus.

Myometrial contractions increase in intensity in the early postpartum period. An increase in intensity is evident, perhaps due to the decreased volume. The high levels of activity diminish smoothly and progressively, plateauing one to two hours postpartum (Hendricks, Eskes, & Saameli, 1972, p. 890). Cell size increases during pregnancy to accommodate uterine contents, so the subsequent process of involution in the puerperium results from decrease in cytoplasm and cell size (Easterling, 1977, p. 708).

The endometrial bed, site of placental attachment, requires days to weeks to reepithelialize (Netter, 1965, p. 121). The site is elevated and irregular after delivery of the placenta. It is composed primarily of thrombosed vascular sinusoids (Easterling, 1977, p. 708). The classic description of the process of regeneration of the endometrium was proposed by Williams and still stands today. He described an exfoliation due to an undermining of the placental site by an ingrowth of endometrial tissue (1931, p. 664). Thus, scarring does not occur and eventually the site is filled in by normal endometrial tissue. Lochia, the vaginal discharge characteristic of the puerperium, consists of tissues sloughed from the necrotic decidua surrounding the placental site as well as blood and fetal debris (lanugo, vernix, and sometimes meconium). Rubra lochia is the name given to the first discharge, which lasts a couple of days, due to the presence of blood from the venous sinuses exposed by delivery of the placenta. Serous lochia is blood stained, thicker, and more mucoid. It consists of leukocytes, erythrocytes, mucus, various microorganisms, and decidual debris. After several more days a transition to alba lochia occurs. This lochia is whitish and creamy and may persist up to six weeks. It is mostly decidual cells, leukocytes, epithelial cells, and other uterine debris, bacteria, mucus, and cholestrin crystals (Greenhill & Friedman, 1974, p. 314). The odor should be earthy and similar to that of menses.

The uterus at delivery weighs about 1,000 grams. After delivery, myometrial contractions cause involution to a level at or below the umbilicus. At this point it is approximately 14 centimeters long, 12 centimeters wide, and 10 centimeters thick (Easterling, 1977, p. 708). The normal shape is globular. At the end of one week, the uterus weighs only 500 grams, and by the end of eight weeks it weighs only 60 to 80 grams (Greenhill & Friedman, 1974, p. 312). Figures 2.1 and 2.2 depict the woman's pelvic anatomy, emphasizing the extensive vascular network.

For several days after delivery, the cervix and lower uterine segment are edematous, thin, and fragile (Easterling, 1977, pp. 708–709). Immediately after delivery it is one centimeter thick and three to six centimeters long. The exocervix may appear ragged and the lateral margins seem to be lacerated, accounting for the slit-like appearance of the parous cervix. The os is dilated three to four centimeters for the first few days, and then closes so that by the end of the second week, it is only a few millimeters (Easterling, 1977, p. 709).

Vagina and Perineum

In the immediate postpartum period, the vagina may be bruised, swollen, sensitive, and sore from the stretching and trauma of the birth process. If an episiotomy has been done or lacerations have occurred, sutures may be in place. Rugae, smoothed by the enlargement and stretching required for delivery, reappear by the end of the fourth week. Until that time, the vagina appears smooth walled. By six to eight

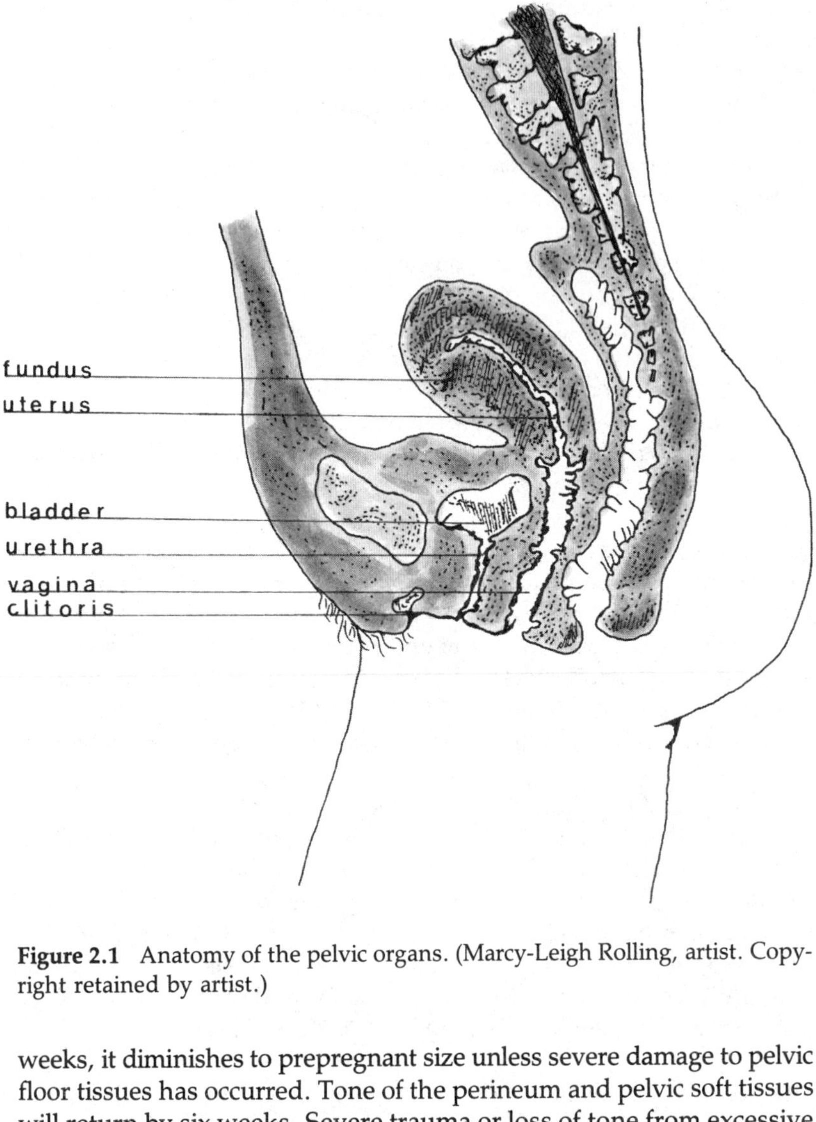

Figure 2.1 Anatomy of the pelvic organs. (Marcy-Leigh Rolling, artist. Copyright retained by artist.)

weeks, it diminishes to prepregnant size unless severe damage to pelvic floor tissues has occurred. Tone of the perineum and pelvic soft tissues will return by six weeks. Severe trauma or loss of tone from excessive stretching for many deliveries may cause a cystocele, rectocele, or urethrocele to occur.

Hemorrhoids may be present as a result of pressure on the perineal area from the fetus or during expulsion, which in turn causes dilatation of veins. A third-degree or fourth-degree laceration extending to or through the anal mucosa and the resulting repair may make the entire perineum tender, swollen, and sore, and predispose to formation of a hematoma.

Perineal or paravaginal hematomas may develop independent of lacerations and are sources of bleeding in addition to an atonic uterus. Lacerations occur anywhere in the birth canal from cervix and vagina through the urethral area and the perineal body and anal ring. Presence of an episiotomy is no assurance of absence of lacerations. Brendsel, Peterson, and Mehl found in their investigation that episiotomies contributed to symptoms and signs of pelvic discomfort and relaxation (1980, p. 49). They state that "routine episiotomy assures some residual sequelae" (p. 59). These authors seem to feel that episiotomies and tears are more or less "equal evils" (p. 59).

Abdomen and Gastrointestinal Tract

Separation of the rectus abdominis muscle, diastasis recti abdominis, is a common occurrence during pregnancy. This condition may persist postpartum and is usually, although not always, associated with

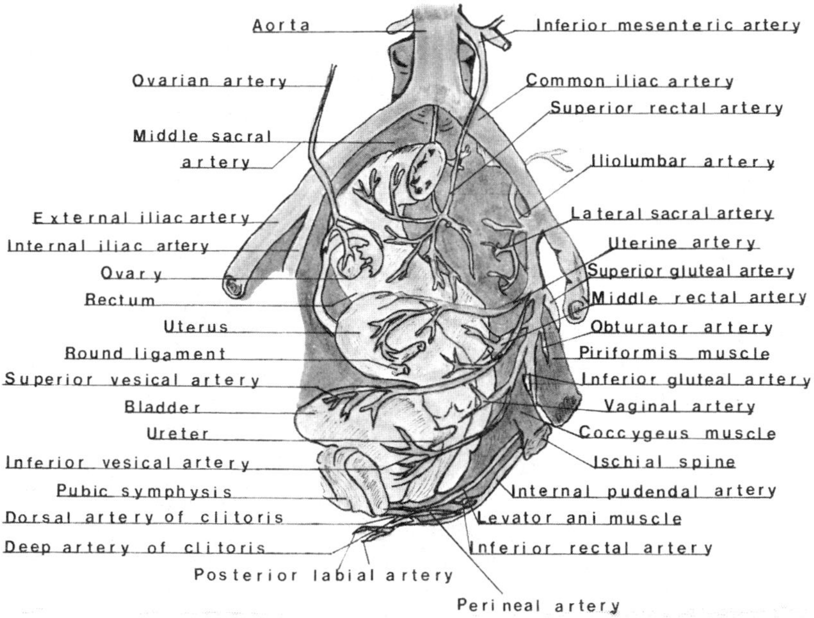

Figure 2.2 Vascular supply to the pelvic organs. (Marcy-Leigh Rolling, artist. Copyright retained by artist.)

multiple pregnancy and polyhydramnios (Easterling, 1977, p. 709). Relaxation of abdominal muscles is common for one to two weeks postpartum and return to a nonparous state requires six to seven weeks. Exercise can restore muscle tone. Although the skin will regain some of its elasticity, some striae will persist. They will turn silvery white with time, but usually will not disappear completely. The linea nigra will fade and often disappear. Return of the umbilicus to its normal inverted state accompanies increase in abdominal muscle tone.

Relieved of pressure of the encroaching uterus, the gastrointestinal tract begins the transition to prepregnancy state and functioning. The decreased motility common to pregnancy resolves rapidly unless the woman has received excess medication or anesthesia. Return to full gastrointestinal functioning is fairly rapid even after a cesarean section. Occasionally paralytic ileus occurs as a complication as in the case of all abdominal surgery. Constipation in the first few days or difficulty in bowel evacuation has several causes or contributing factors: diet, fluid intake, persistent decreased motility, lax abdominal muscles, diastasis recti abdominis, decreased activity or exercise, sore episiotomy, hemorrhoids, and third- or fourth-degree laceration. Delay in evacuation for three or four days postpartum may be related to any of the foregoing and, in addition, to administration of an enema and the period of fasting required during labor or prior to and after cesarean section. Resolution of food intolerances and indigestion experienced during pregnancy resolves when anatomical position and mechanical and physiologic function of the gastrointestinal tract are restored.

Urinary Tract

The frequency of urination which accompanies descent of the presenting part resolves with delivery unless cystitis occurs. Trauma to the bladder and urethra from forceps or the presenting part can occur. Diminution of bladder tone and detrusor reflex can result from trauma and/or effects of anesthesia. Urethral spasm is related to trauma or referred pain from a tender episiotomy. The bladder may be bruised and/or urethra swollen secondary to trauma. Lacerations into the uretheral orifice can occur. Bladder tone and sensation may be absent and bladder distention so great that it is palpable above the symphysis and displacing the uterus up and to the right. This process can contribute to uterine atony and resultant hemorrhage. Loss of tone and sensation can also lead to urinary retention, stasis, and infection. The bladder may be injured during cesarean section, necessitating surgical repair and prolongation of a continuous indwelling catheter until healing is complete. In its position overlying the lower segment of the pregnant uterus, the bladder is particularly vulnerable when a low flap or extraperitoneal cesarean is done.

Twenty-four to 48 hours after delivery, the woman will experience diuresis. This is the result of the body's effort to unload fluid accumulated during pregnancy. Fluid retention secondary to the sodium-retaining properties of the progesterones accounts for a portion of the weight gain during pregnancy. Diuresis is a normal phenomenon and part of the process of restoration (Hawkins & Higgins, 1981, p. 391).

Cardiovascular and Respiratory Systems

Cardiac output, which increases during labor, peaks sometime during the puerperium. One study demonstrated levels 60 and 80 percent above those prior to labor. A few minutes after delivery, output is 40 to 50 percent above prelabor and declines to prepregnancy levels in two to three weeks (Ueland & Hansen, 1969, p. 8). Alterations in stroke volume account for these changes, as does a decrease in heart rate (Easterling, 1977, p. 710).

Blood volume loss at 60 minutes postpartum averages 10.2 percent for vaginal deliveries and 17.4 percent for cesarean section. There is a steady decline over the first three days of the puerperium to a mean of 16.2 percent for both groups. The blood volume is stable from 60 minutes postpartum to the fifth day in women who have had cesarean sections. It declines to the third day in women who have delivered vaginally. At six weeks postpartum, there is no difference in blood volume between the two groups of women, but the hematocrit is lower in women who have had cesarean sections (Ueland, 1976, p. 671).

Once birth occurs, the uterus descends in the peritoneal cavity and the diaphragm is restored to its normal position. The cardiac axis thus returns to normal and electrocardiographic features are normalized as well (Easterling, 1977, p. 710). Compression of lungs and compromise of respiratory function by impingement of the uterus on the diaphragm ceases and normal respiratory function is restored.

Vital signs. Hypertension in the puerperium results from toxemia, continuation of preexisting chronic hypertensive condition, or the effects of ergonovine maleate or methylergonovine maleate administration immediately postpartum. Hypotension may be due to excessive blood loss or the effects of regional anesthesia.

Temperature elevation in the first 24 hours is the result of the dramatic hormonal changes, dehydration, and fatigue. After 24 hours, infection is the primary cause.

The pulse rate may be unusually low following delivery. Although a definitive cause has not been isolated, suspicion is directed toward a multifactional approach. Rapid pulse is usually associated with hemorrhage.

Iron deficiency anemia. Anemia occurs because of the demands of the fetus for iron over the last month of gestation and as a result of excessive blood loss. It is common to do a hematocrit and hemoglobin in the early puerperium to determine whether anemia is present.

Resumption of Menstruation

Reestablishment of regular, ovulatory cycles after pregnancy is a complex phenomenon. For women who are not breast feeding, menses resume by 6 weeks postpartum for 40 percent, 12 weeks for 65 percent, and 24 weeks for 90 percent. About 50 percent of these cycles are anovulatory (Vorherr, 1974). Only 15 percent of women who are breast feeding resume menses by 6 weeks and only 45 percent by 12 weeks. As many as 80 percent of these women have one or more anovulatory cycles before ovulation occurs (Vorherr, 1974). In one study, the mean period of lactation amenorrhea was found to be 14.6 months for women who only breast-fed their infants (Jelliffe & Jelliffe, 1979, p. 50). Martinez and Nalezienski found that between 1979 and 1978, 46.6 percent of women were breast feeding while in hospital; when the infant was two months of age, 34.9 percent were still breast feeding, 26.8 percent at four months, and 20.5 percent at five to six months (1979, p. 688). Prolactin appears to inhibit gonadotropins, which in turn reduces ovarian steroid production and produces physiologic amenorrhea (Easterling, 1977, p. 711). Since it can be demonstrated that the pituitary is insensitive to synthetic luteinizing hormone releasing factor (LRE) regardless of mode of infant feeding, inhibition may occur in the hypothalamus (LeMaire et al., 1974, p. 916).

Resumption of menses, therefore, may or may not be preceded by ovulation and ovulatory cycles may occur even with lactation. Ovulation may precede resumption of menstruation, so conception may be possible as early as a few weeks after giving birth.

Sexuality. The muscle tone of the perineal area requires time for restoration. Presence of an episiotomy or lacerations make the perineal area tender and sore. Diminution of estrogen following delivery of the placenta and influences of oxytocin and prolactin during lactation cause the vaginal mucosa to lubricate less profusely. Breasts may be tender, and leaking of milk can contribute to discomfort. Women may feel guilt and role conflict in being both mothers and sexual beings. Alterations in body shape, body image, and loss of control over body functions may make the woman feel unattractive (Derthick, 1974, p. 509). On the other hand, feelings of eroticism and sexuality may actually increase for the woman who is breast-feeding.

Breasts

Mammary glands in the human are composed of 15 to 20 lobes connecting with ducts through breast tissue to converge on the nipple or papilla. Lobes divide into lobules and acini (or alveoli). Ducts dilate to become ampullae before they converge on the nipple and these, in turn, send many minute ducts to open in the nipple. The pigmented areola surrounds the nipple. The nipple is generally erectile due to the contraction of muscle fibers. The base of nipple and areola have numerous sebaceous glands. These may enlarge during lactation and appear as tubercles. The function is to secrete a fatty substance to protect the nipple during sucking. Washing breasts with soap is drying because it removes this natural protection.

The breasts themselves are usually cone-like in shape, the left often slightly larger than the right (Gray, 1974, p. 1038). Asymmetry is normal and no cause for alarm. Breasts consist of glandular tissue, fibrous tissue which connects the lobes, and adipose tissue between lobes.

Blood to the breasts is supplied by thoracic branches of the axillary, intercostals, and internal mammary arteries. Veins form an "anastomotic circle" (Gray, 1901, p. 1040) around the nipple, and blood is then transmitted to the axillary and internal mammary veins. The lymphatic system borders the lower margin of the pectoralis major and thus to axillary nodes. Figure 2.3 illustrates the venous and lymphatic configuration of the breast. A few axillary nodes run along the inner margin of the breast and empty into anterior mediastinal glands. Nerve supply comes from the anterior and lateral cutaneous nerves of the thorax (Gray, 1901, pp. 1039–1040; Townsend, 1980, pp. 5–6). The breasts are not quiescent during pregnancy. Under the influences of progesterones and estrogens of pregnancy, breasts increase in size and colostrum may be produced. Prolactin levels rise during pregnancy and may play a role in the increase in breast size. So do insulin and human placental lactogen (HPL). All of these decline dramatically after delivery to or below prepregnancy levels (Easterling, 1977, p. 710). Nonetheless, three to five days after delivery, milk production begins and breasts become engorged. Prolactin levels increase in surges and seem to have some influence on initiation of milk production. The greatest influence of all, however, seems to be sucking. The mechanism seems to involve tac-

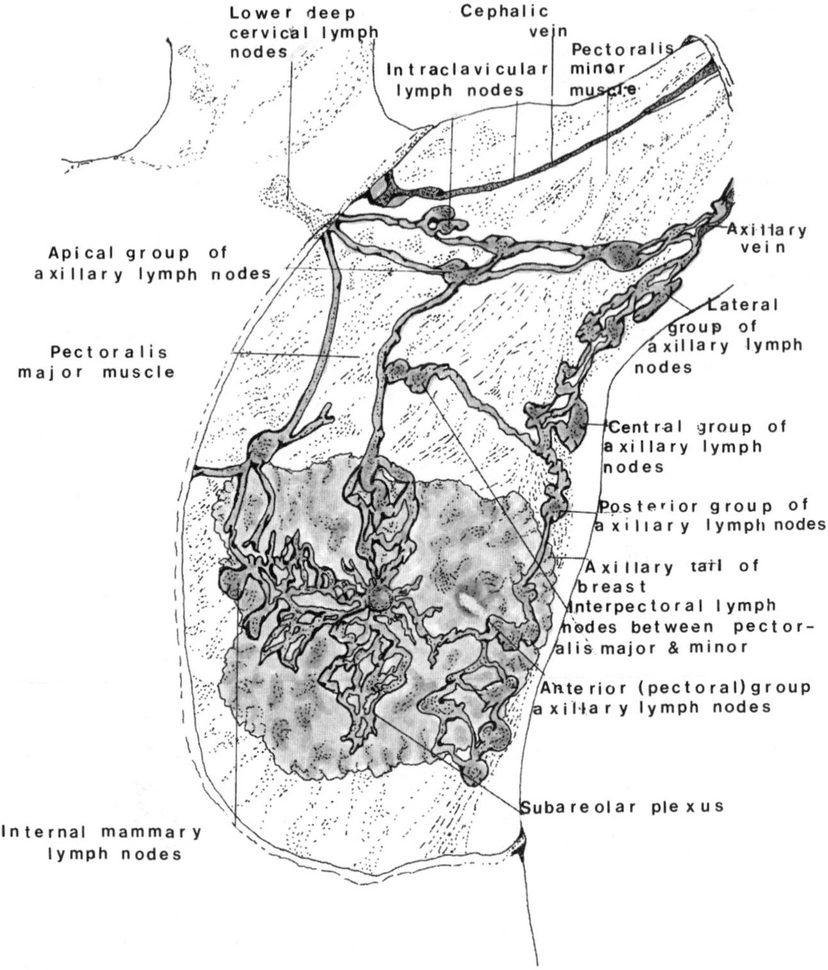

Figure 2.3 Vascular and lymphatic supply of the breast. (Marcy-Leigh Rolling, artist. Copyright retained by artist.)

tile nerve endings in the areola which, it is hypothesized, transmit a stimulus to the nuclei of the hypothalamus. That stimulus, in turn, causes an increase in synthesis and transport of oxytocin to the posterior pituitary whence it passes into the circulation. Oxytocin is known to stimulate the myoepithelial cells surrounding the alveoli and ducts to contract, and thus milk is ejected from the nipple. This is called the "let down" reflex (Easterling, 1977, p. 710). An infant crying may also stimulate this "let down" of milk. Because oxytocins cause contraction of smooth muscle, nursing an infant will cause the uterus to contract. Thus, putting an infant to breast right after delivery is beneficial in promoting involution. Oxytocin seems to play little role in milk production. Prolactin appears to be the important hormone for milk supply, stimulating the epithelium of the alveoli. Stimulation of the nipple causes a message to be sent to the hypothalamus wherein prolactin-inhibiting factor is suppressed (Easterling, 1977, p. 710). It can be demonstrated that, after a few weeks of nursing, prolactin levels decline. The most important factors in sustaining milk supply seem to be sucking and presence of the infant. Fluid intake is also a critical component, as is the woman's nutritional state. Figure 2.4 illustrates the anatomy of the breast.

In the past, women who did not wish to breast-feed routinely received synthetic estrogen products in an effort to suppress lactation. With the advent of concern for the safety of estrogen-containing drugs, informed consent was sought before these preparations were administered. Efforts are now directed toward development of drugs which might achieve the same results without the hazards of estrogen. Bromocriptine mesylate (Parlodel®) has recently been touted as an effective, nonhormonal, nonestrogenic suppressant for postpartum lactation. Interestingly, the course of therapy is 14 days. If no nursing occurs, natural suppression of lactation will normally take place within that time frame, so the cost/benefit ratio must be examined closely. Other nonchemical methods of discouraging milk production and engorgement will be discussed in Chapters 3 and 6.

At termination of lactation, involution of the breasts occurs and occupies a period of about three months. Decrease in size is the major change, unlike the loss in lobular-alveolar components which accompanies menopause. Breast size rarely returns to that of a prepregnant state, but is generally larger (Townsend, 1980, p. 8). Persistence of discharge after the infant has been weaned suggests continued stimulation or pathology and should be assessed. Resumption of regular breast examination after menses should be encouraged once weaning is completed. Breast examination will be discussed in Chapter 6.

Risk Factors

Major risk factors to the woman during the puerperium which may lead to crisis include hemorrhage, infections, eclampsia, venous disease, depression, and psychosis. Inability to establish an adequate milk supply for the infant's demands is one risk associated with lactation.

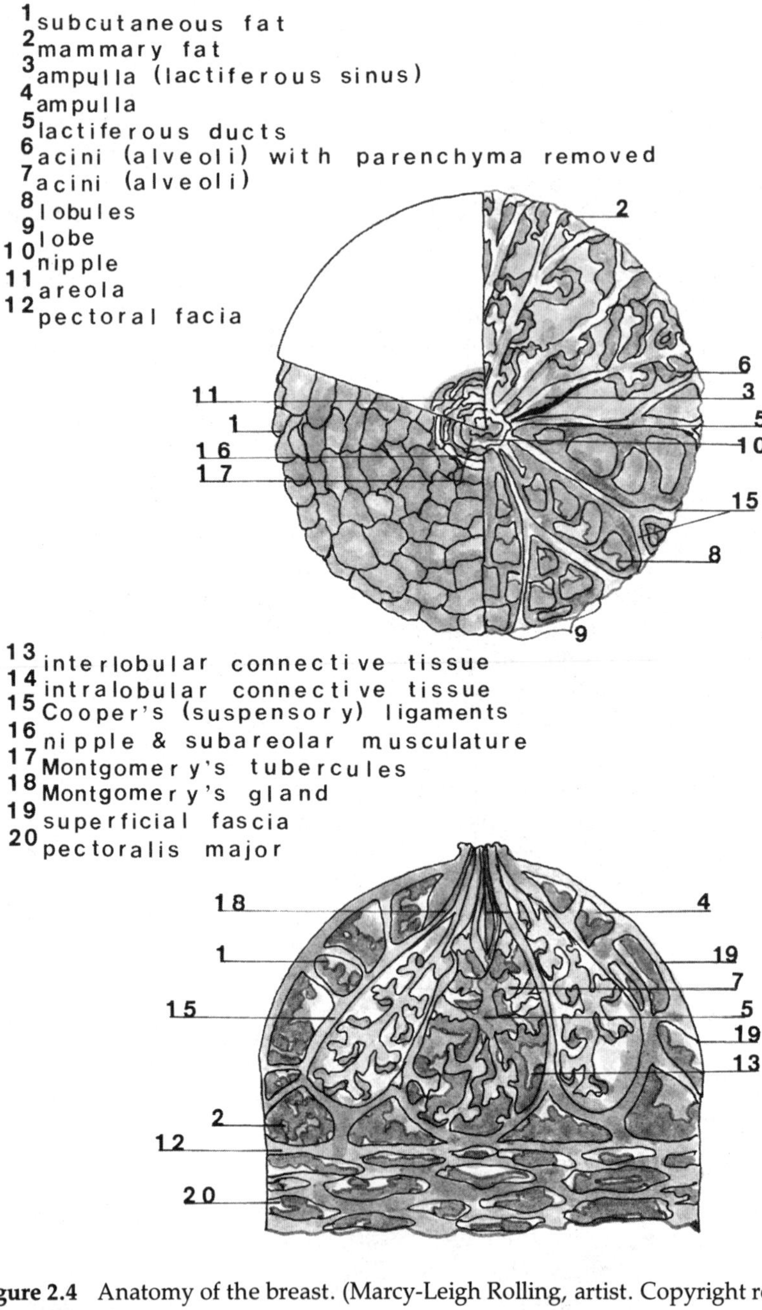

Figure 2.4 Anatomy of the breast. (Marcy-Leigh Rolling, artist. Copyright retained by artist.)

Mastitis also occurs, usually in association with breast feeding. Risks to the woman will be discussed in detail in Chapter 4.

Adaptation of the Infant to Extrauterine Life

The abrupt descent of the infant into the world-at-large disturbs the relative calm and equilibrium experienced during gestation. Accustomed to a relatively stable temperature in the amniotic sac, bathed in the soothing warm fluid, comforted by the woman's heartbeat, the infant is suddenly thrust into a cool, noisy environment replete with stimuli. Adaptation to extrauterine life must occur rapidly if the infant is to survive. If crisis occurs in that adaptation process, prompt interventions must be instituted to restore equilibrium and support adaptive processes.

Respiratory System

Respirations are initiated by cold, light, noise, gravity, pain, hypercapnia, respiratory acidosis, and hypoxia (Gimbel & Nocon, 1977, pp. 11–15). Although human fetuses are known through observation with ultrasound and fetoscopy to "practice" breathing in utero, breathing now is vital to exchange of gases. Dependence upon the marvelous exchange made possible by the placenta ends at birth. Sufficient amounts of surfactant (phospholipids) must be present to maintain expansion of the alveoli so that they do not collapse between inspirations. Respiratory movements of the newborn are generally diaphragmatic. Expansion of both lungs should occur rapidly with initiation of breathing and occasional grunts and rales should disappear within the first hour after birth.

Circulation

At birth, the fetal circulatory pattern is no longer necessary. Immediate circulatory changes are imperative in order to move blood through the lungs.

Changes in pressure in the lungs and chambers of the heart during the first few minutes after birth cause the fetal structures to close. Blood returning to the heart from the lungs via the pulmonary veins increases pressure in the left atrium, causing the foramen ovale to close. Lowered pulmonary resistance, resulting from expansion of the lungs, causes the pressure in the pulmonary artery to decrease. Increased aortic pressure then causes reverse blood flow in the ductus arteriosus. This small vessel constricts within three to four days and by two months is closed by fibrotic tissue (Whaley & Wong, 1979, pp. 250–251). The ductus venosus closes also at birth and eventually becomes a ligament.

Gastrointestinal Tract

During tenure in the uterus, the fetus swallows amniotic fluid. At birth, the intestines normally contain a significant amount of sterile material known as meconium. Usually the first meconium stool is passed within 24 hours after birth. Meconium is composed of amniotic fluid, fetal hair, fetal epithelium, vernix, lanugo, and bile residues. Shortly after birth, the intestines will begin to distend with air as the infant swallows.

The infant is capable of digestion of an unsophisticated sort at birth. Stomach capacity of a full-term neonate is approximately 90 milliliters. Emptying time is rapid, somewhere between two and a half and three hours, and peristalsis active. Because of this, the newborn may have a bowel movement as often as with every feeding (Whaley & Wong, 1979, p. 257). Small stomach capacity at birth is compensated for by rapid emptying, assuring that the infant will be able to handle a daily volume of feedings sufficient to needs for growth and maintenance.

Genitourinary Tract

The fetus swallows amniotic fluid and urinates in utero. One of the major components of amniotic fluid is fetal urine. Urination normally occurs within the first few minutes or hours after birth, certainly by 24 hours. The kidneys are not yet fully mature, so their capacity to concentrate urine is not refined. Normal output is 200 to 300 milliliters by seven days of age. Since the bladder empties when 15 milliliters of urine are present, the infant may appear to be voiding constantly.

Nervous System

The nervous system of the newborn is immature at birth. Reflexes necessary for survival are present in the full-term infant: rooting, sucking, and swallowing. The infant can see, hear, smell, and taste, allowing considerable interaction with the environment. Tactile sensation, too, is present, and the infant is highly responsive to touch. Brazelton emphasizes the importance of the infant's capacity to interact with and act upon his or her environment. His assessment scale focuses on the infant's behavioral responses (1973). Infants from birth demonstrate variations in state. They also are individual in their irritability, threshold for stimuli, and circadian rhythms. The extremely versatile infant by the third week usually adapts to adult-like circadian regularity (Deters, 1980, p. 250). Their interactional capacities allow them to respond to, but also to control to a degree, their environments. The infant should demonstrate the entire range of normal infant states: regular sleep, active rapid eye movement (REM) sleep, quiet wakefulness, active wakefulness, fussing, crying, and indeterminate state (Binzley, 1977, pp. 102–103). Thoman's work on the social responsiveness of infants emphasizes the social capacities of the newborn and the marvelous adaptive qualities of infants. Her longitudinal studies of mother–infant pairs indicates the reciprocity of which infants are capable in their adaptation to extrauterine life (Thoman, 1978, pp. 50–54; Trotter, 1980, pp. 234–235).

Musculoskeletal System

The full-term infant, confined in the close quarters of the uterus, is released at birth. In response to the deluge of stimuli birth presents him or her with, the infant maintains or returns to the fetal position in order to calm himself or herself and regain control. Capable of a limited range of gross motor activities, the infant utilizes these in signaling and contacting the environment. Some of the primitive reflexes present at birth represent interplay between nervous and musculoskeletal systems: rooting, sucking, swallowing, grasping. Very rapidly the infant adopts self-comforting measures: hitching up to the corner of the bassinette or crib, sucking on thumb or fingers. The ability to lift the head even momentarily off the mattress allows the infant to change head position from side to side. Attempts at head control are already present at birth and the infant works to improve abilities. An infant in the awake state is generally very active, signaling readiness to begin the process of adaptation to and exploration of the extrauterine world.

Risk Factors

The neonate is at risk in adaptation to extrauterine life. Primary risks in the adaptive processes include respiratory distress, cardiovascular insufficiency, failure to pass urine or meconium in the first 24 hours, cold stress and hypothermia, metabolic interruptions, hematologic conditions, and infection. These risks are the result of maladaptation caused by anomalies, immaturity of organ systems, external events such as birth trauma or maternal disease, and/or failure of normal adaptive mechanisms such as closure of the foramen ovale and ductus arteriosus. Nursing interventions for infants at risk will be discussed in Chapter 7.

Summary

Biophysical adaptation immediately after birth is complex and essential for both the woman and her infant. Failure to adapt to a nonpregnant state can lead to crisis for the woman. The infant whose adaptive responses to extrauterine life are insufficient may experience crises such as respiratory or cardiovascular distress. Helping the woman and her infant to remain in a precrisis state requires close assessment of adaptation, and augmentation if the individual's coping mechanisms are insufficient. The chapters to follow will discuss nursing aspects of the care of women and their infants during the puerperium.

References

Binzley, V. State: overlooked factor in newborn nursing. *American Journal of Nursing*, 1977, *77*, 102–103.

Brazelton, T. B. *Neonatal behavioral assessment scale*. National Spastics Monograph No. 50. London: Heinemann & Son, 1973.

Brendsel, C., Peterson, G., & Mehl, L. E. Routine episiotomy and pelvic symptomatology. *Women & Health*, 1980, *5*(4), 49–60.

Danforth, D. W., & Hendricks, C. H. Physiology of uterine action. In D. N. Danforth (Ed.), *Obstetrics and gynecology* (3rd ed.). Hagerstown, Md.: Harper & Row, 1977, pp. 522–564.

Derthick, N. Sexuality in pregnancy and the puerperium. *Birth and the Family Journal*, 1974, *1*(4), 5–9.

Deters, G. E. Circadian rhythm phenomenon. *The American Journal of Maternal Child Nursing*, 1980, *5*(4), 249–251.

Easterling, W. E. The puerperium. In D. W. Danforth (Ed.), *Obstetrics and gynecology* (3rd ed.). Hagerstown, Md.: Harper & Row, 1977, pp. 708–721.

Gimbel, J., & Nocon, J. J. The physiological basis for the Leboyer approach to childbirth. *Journal of Obstetric, Gynecologic, and Neonatal Nursing*, 1977, *6*(1), 11–15.

Gray, H. *Anatomy, descriptive and surgical* (1901 ed.). Philadelphia: Running Press, 1974.

Greenhill, J. P., & Friedman, E. A. *Biological principles and modern practice of obstetrics*. Philadelphia: W. B. Saunders, 1974.

Hawkins, J. W., & Higgins, L. P. *Maternity and gynecologic nursing: Women's health care*. Philadelphia: J. B. Lippincott, 1981.

Hendricks, C. H., Eskes, T. K. A. B., & Saameli, K. Uterine contractability at delivery and in the puerperium. *American Journal of Obstetrics and Gynecology*, 1972, *83*.

Jelliffe, D. B., & Jelliffe, E. P. P. Postpartum amenorrhea: hormones versus nutrition. *Birth and the Family Journal*, 1979, *6*(1), 49–50.

Kumaresan, P., Anandarangam, P. B., Dianzon, W., & Vasicka, A. Plasma oxytocin levels during human pregnancy and labor as determined by radioimmunoassay. *American Journal of Obstetrics and Gynecology*, 1974, *119*(2), 215–223.

LeMaire, J. W., Shipiro, A. G., Riggal, F., & Nst Yang. Temporary pituitary insensitivity to stimulation by synthetic LRF during the postpartum period. *Journal of Clinical Endocrinology and Metabolism*, 1974, *38*.

Martinez, G. A., & Nalezienski, J. P. The recent trend in breast feeding. *Pediatrics*, 1979, *64*(5), 686–692.

Netter, F. H. *The Ciba collection of medical illustrations, Vol. 2, Reproductive system*. Summit, N.J.: Ciba, 1965.

Thoman, E. B. Ontogeny of the mother-infant relationship. In S. Trotter & E. B. Thoman (Eds.), *Social responsiveness of infants*. Johnson & Johnson, 1978.

Townsend, C. M. Breast lumps. *Clinical Symposia*, 1980, *32*(2). Summit, N.J.: Ciba, 1980.

Trotter, R. J. Born too soon. *Science News*, 1980, *118*(15), 234–235.

Ueland, K. Maternal cardiovascular dynamics. VII. Intrapartum blood volume changes. *American Journal of Obstetrics and Gynecology*, 1976, *126*(6), 671–677.

Ueland, K., & Hansen, J. M. Maternal and cardiovascular dynamics. III. Labor and delivery under local and caudal anesthesia. *American Journal of Obstetrics and Gynecology*, 1969, *103*.

Vorherr, H. *The breast*. New York: Academic Press, 1974.

Whaley, L. F., & Wong, D. L. *Nursing care of infants and children*. St. Louis: C. V. Mosby, 1979.

Williams, J. W. Regeneration of the uterine mucosa after delivery with especial reference to the placental site. *American Journal of Obstetrics and Gynecology*, 1931, *22*.

3

Immediate Postpartum Assessment, Nursing Augmentation, and Intervention

Introduction

During the first hours postpartum, Rising (1974) suggests that there are three critical questions that must be answered: will the blood pressure stabilize; will the uterus clamp down; and will diuresis begin? Equally important are the questions parents ask themselves: do we have enough love; can we afford a (another) child; have we prepared the other children? (p. 870). The puerperium represents a time in a woman's life with a high potential for crisis. The caring and support she receives from nurses is critical to her well-being, both biophysical and psychosocial. This chapter will address the immediate postpartum needs of women and how best nurses may augment the women's own coping mechanisms to avert crisis.

Assessment for Risk Factors

The first hour after delivery is often called the fourth stage of labor. It is during this critical time that most biophysical complications occur. This is also a time when initiation of attachment between woman and infant should be encouraged, if at all possible. Nursing augmentation should be based on continuous assessment of vital signs, involution, and the adjustments the woman is making in her assumption of a new role as well as the infant's social behaviors and adaptation to extrauterine life.

For the first hour, and perhaps longer, the woman and her infant will be under close observation in the birthing room, delivery room, or a recovery area. Transfer to postpartum rarely occurs until the woman's condition has stabilized for at least one hour. Once transfer is accomplished, the woman and her infant become the responsibility of the postpartum nurses. Ideally, the dyad are assigned to one nurse. Some institutions, however, have chosen to retain the more traditional pattern of nursery and postpartum nurses, so that the woman is transferred to the care of a nurse on the postpartum unit and the infant is usually taken, at least temporarily, to the newborn nursery area. Chapter 8 is an extensive discussion of implementation of family-centered maternity care.

The woman is very vulnerable immediately after delivery. Having experienced a very emotional and physically stressful event which heralds a role transition to parenthood, she now finds herself transferred to an unfamiliar part of the maternity unit and is faced with a new set of caregivers. Routines of assessment and care may be unfamiliar as well. If her infant has been taken to the nursery, she may be disappointed at the disruption in the attachment process. At the same time, she may crave sleep, food, relief from discomfort, and attention to her needs. What may seem routine to experienced nurses can be frightening, uncomfortable, and intrusive to a woman who finds herself the passive recipient of postpartum care. Nurses who care for women and their infants have a special challenge. Caring for must be balanced with caring about and with, as the woman assumes responsibility for her own care and that of her infant. How the woman perceives the caring she receives will affect her ability to parent and her self-image as a woman and a mother.

History

A brief pregnancy and intrapartal history is important to the nurse assuming responsibility for care of a woman in the postpartum unit. Polyhydramnios, multiple pregnancy, a history as a grandmultipara or of previous postpartum hemorrhage, or desultory or prolonged labor all increase the risk of postpartum hemorrhage. A history of cesarean delivery, placenta previa, abruptio placenta, retained placenta or placental fragments, a traumatic delivery, large baby, toxemia, oxytocin induction, and excessive blood loss in this or previous delivery experiences places the woman at greater risk for postpartum complications. It is important to know whether the woman has any medical conditions such as diabetes, hypertension, cardiac disease, multiple sclerosis, or carcinoma, whether she smokes, and whether she has a history of drug or alcohol abuse. If the infant is transferred to and cared for in the nursery, a report on the child's condition is essential to giving the woman holistic care. Finally, any special cultural traditions or rites should be noted (Clark, 1978).

Vital Signs

It is customary to check the woman's vital signs every half hour to every hour for the first three to four hours after delivery. Most postpartum units establish protocols which allow some flexibility for individual cases. Physician's routines exist, but are probably less useful than the assessment and decisions of the nurse caring for the woman.

Since blood volume increases substantially during pregnancy for uterine perfusion and in preparation for labor and delivery, significant blood loss can occur before it is reflected in vital signs. The fall in blood pressure and rise in pulse which are the results of hemorrhage may, thus, be precipitous rather than gradual. Hypertension is usually due to ergonovine maleate or methylergonovine maleate, but may signal impending eclampsia, with or without a history of preeclampsia during pregnancy. Hypertension due to the aforementioned causes may also mask hemorrhage, so assessment must include evaluation of the uterus and lochia flow. Compare blood pressure readings with those during labor, pregnancy, and, if possible, a prepregnant baseline. The normal range for an individual is a more important base with which to measure change than any so-called norms.

Pulse rate is usually low after delivery. The cause is unknown, most probably multifactorial. A low pulse is considered one index of well-being. A rapid pulse is associated with hemorrhage.

Respiratory rate should be within the range of normal for adults. Increased rate and depth of respiration occur with hemorrhage as a compensatory mechanism. A severe shock state results in shallow, irregular respirations (Thompson, 1978, pp. 37–39).

Temperature elevation in the first 24 hours postpartum is generally due to fatigue, hormonal changes, and/or dehydration. Elevations after 24 hours are usually related to infection.

Thirst is a common symptom of hemorrhage due to loss of blood volume. The increased serum level of sodium which precedes shock due to action of aldosterone and glucocorticoids on the kidneys may also cause thirst. It is important to recognize this symptom and to ascertain whether the woman received any medications that cause drying of mucus membranes (Thompson, 1978, p. 36).

Reproductive Organs

Involution begins immediately after delivery. The uterine fundus can be palpated at approximately the level of the umbilicus for the first 12 to 24 hours, and descends at a rate of one to two centimeters (one finger breadth) daily until it is no longer palpable above the symphysis. The uterus should be firmly contracted and midline. Deviation upward and to the right is caused by a distended bladder. Uterine atony results in hemorrhage, so frequent assessment is necessary to ascertain that the uterus remains firmly contracted and involutes normally. Assessment every one half to one hour for the first several hours in the postpartum unit and then daily until discharge is fairly common protocol. If the uterus is not firmly contracted, massage can be instituted. One hand can be used to massage the fundus and assess for contraction while the other hand guards over the symphysis to prevent inverting the uterus. Before attempting to express clots or debris, it is important to massage the uterus so it will contract. These processes can be painful to the woman, as the uterus, ligaments, and pelvic soft tissues are very sensitive immediately after the trauma of delivery. Excessive manipulation or stimulation of the uterus can cause exhaustion of the muscles and, consequently, atony. The process of involution is illustrated in Figure 3.1.

The woman may experience afterpains, painful contractions of the uterus which promote involution. Afterpains are especially notable in women who are multigravidous, those who have experienced any overdistention of the uterus due to multiple gestation, a very large baby, or hydramnios, those who have received methylergonovine, pitocin, or ergonovine maleate, and those who are breast feeding. These women need reassurance that this is a normal phenomenon. Analgesics, ambulation, and a prone position in bed are other comfort measures.

Lochia flow may peak at 8 to 12 hours after delivery due to increased activity and healing, and then decline. Except for the first few hours after delivery, clots are considered abnormal and should be investigated as to cause. Bleeding over time is important to assess as well as volume. A slow, steady trickle over many hours can lead to shock. Pad counts, saturation, presence and size of clots, and color (bright versus dark red) are all indicators of the amount of blood loss. During the first day or two, a gush of blood is common when the woman gets up after a prolonged period of rest in a horizontal position. Otherwise,

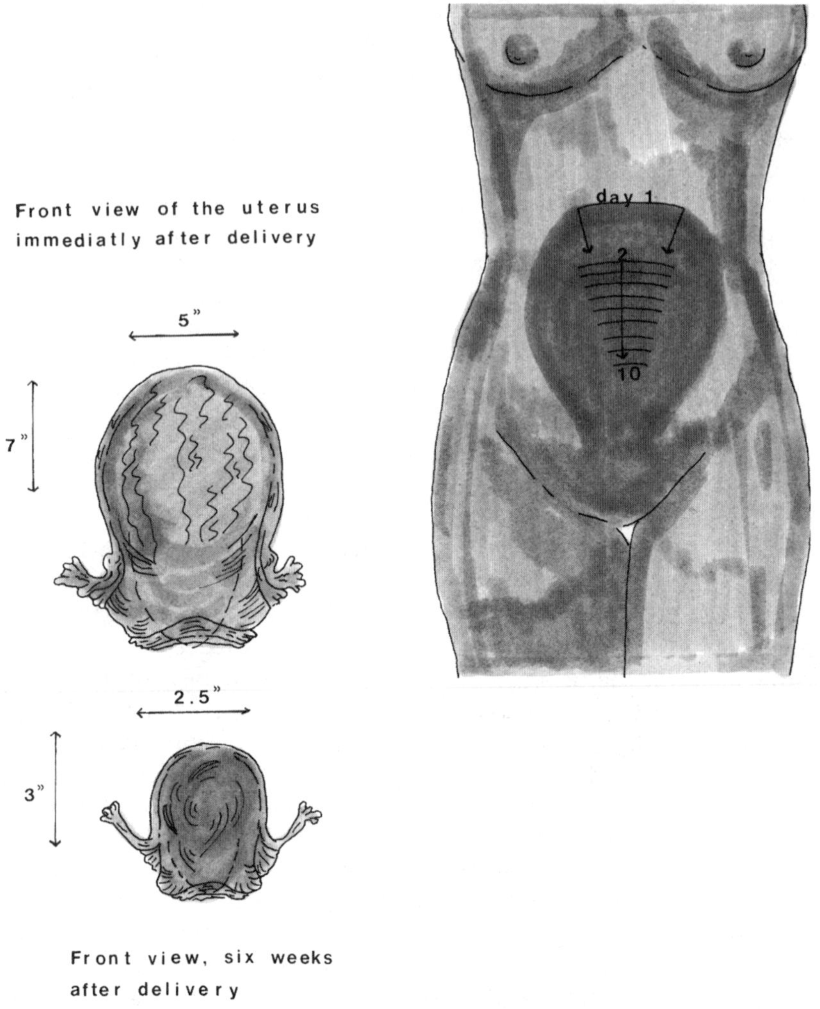

Figure 3.1 Involution of the pelvic organs. (Marcy-Leigh Rolling, artist. Copyright retained by artist.)

bleeding should be moderate, tapering to a scant flow at the end of one week, following a pattern similar to the diminution of menstrual flow.

The vagina and perineum may be sore, bruised, and swollen. Lacerations or an episiotomy may also make the perineum tender. Assessment of healing should be done frequently in the first few hours after delivery and at least daily until discharge. The possibility of a hematoma should not be overlooked if the perineal area is unusually swollen, tender, and/or discolored.

Relief of discomfort is important to the woman's sense of well-being. Application of cold in the first hours after delivery through a cold pack, ice pack, or ice glove can help to minimize swelling. Heat increases circulation and, thus, promotes healing. Sitz baths, hot packs, a warm face cloth, perineal lamps, and warm showers are all good sources of heat.

Early ambulation increases circulation, prevents stasis of lochia, and in addition helps to prevent thrombophlebitis and stasis of respiratory secretions.

Topical anesthetic sprays are used for episiotomy pain and are perceived by some women as helpful. A rubber or plastic inflatable ring or doughnut will displace pressure off the episiotomy site when the woman sits. Teach the woman to squeeze her buttocks together before she sits if she has a medium episiotomy to relieve pressure and pain. Various analgesics are prescribed for perineal discomfort. Salicylates and narcotics are commonly used, as are various nonnarcotic prescription analgesic products.

Pelvic floor exercises (Kegel) will increase soft tissue tone and blood supply, decrease pain, and assist healing (Polden, 1975, p. 57). These exercises are initiated by contracting the muscles of the pelvic floor during urination until the stream stops completely then releasing and contracting alternately until the bladder is empty. Once muscle control is mastered, the exercises may be done at times other than during urination. Often women are taught these exercises during preparation for childbirth classes.

Persistent bright red bleeding in the presence of a firmly contracted uterus that is midline and involuting normally suggests lacerations of the birth canal or formation of a hematoma. If inspection of the perineum and vulva does not reveal a source of bleeding and there is no hematoma visible, speculum examination may need to be done in the operating room to locate the source of bleeding and ligate or repair it. Lacerations of the cervix and vagina as well as hematoma formation in the broad ligament are the most common sources of hemorrhage after uterine atony.

Perineal care is done in a variety of ways in different institutions, but the principles are the same. Women are encouraged to cleanse the vulvar area in some way each time they urinate or move their bowels. Cleansing may be done with special solutions and cotton balls, prepared perineal wipes, and plastic squirt bottles filled with warm water. Some institutions recommend showers once or twice a day for cleansing or sitz baths. These are but a few methods that may be used.

Women may need to be taught to wipe from front to back to avoid *Escherichia coli* contamination and to apply perineal pads in the same manner.

Abdomen and Gastrointestinal Tract

Abdominal musculature may be lax after delivery. Early ambulation helps to restore muscle tone and also prevent constipation. So does gradual resumption of exercise. The intestines and stomach return to their normal positions after delivery. Appetite varies from woman to woman. Some women are not hungry right after delivery; some are ravenous. The availability of food and fluids on a maternity unit should be assured 24 hours a day so those women who are hungry can be fed. Oral fluid intake needs to be initiated as soon as possible after delivery in order to compensate for loss through sweat, urine, and lochia and lack of fluids during labor. Bowel evacuation may be delayed until three or four days after delivery because of stretched abdominal musculature and loss of tone, lack of food in labor, admission enema, and fear of damage or pain related to hemorrhoids and the episiotomy. Diet contributes in an important way to resumption of normal bowel hygiene. Fiber, bulk, and fluids are necessary, as well as exercise.

Hemorrhoids often occur during pregnancy and/or labor and delivery, especially during expulsion. Ointments and anesthetic sprays, sitz baths, warm packs, dry heat, witch hazel compresses, ice packs, and analgesics are common relief measures. Diet teaching is important to prevent constipation. Stool softeners or cathartics are often given postpartum to make the first bowel movement easier. Pelvic floor exercises also help healing and diminish pain. Cathartics appear in breast milk, so women who are breast feeding must rely on other measures to reduce difficulties with bowel evacuation.

Breast Care

Breasts should be inspected for cracks or fissures in the nipples and for engorgement. When the milk "comes in" on day two or three, breasts may become hard, painful, and warm to the touch with prominent veins and lobes palpable as hard lumps. Transient temperature elevation is said to occur in some women associated with engorgement, but infection should be ruled out.

A supportive bra or breast binder helps to relieve engorgement and to provide support. Breast care includes daily shower (no soap), and a lanolin-base cream to prevent drying and cracking of nipples. Ice can help to relieve engorgement for women who are not nursing.

Brooten and colleagues in their investigation compared four methods of intervention to prevent and control engorgement and pain in women who had chosen to bottle feed their infants. They found that bromocriptine mesylate caused women to experience less engorgement, pain, and leaking than any other treatment. A compression binder was helpful in diminishing leaking and was useful in causing pain to subside more rapidly. On the first and second postpartum days, the women were relatively free from breast pain, and engorgement had not yet occurred. The nonpharmacologic treatments (ice, fluid restriction, and compression binder) resulted in the most pain and leaking on days three, four, five, and six (1983, pp. 228–229).

Urinary Tract

The bladder may be bruised, the urethra swollen, and either may be damaged by forceps or pounding of the presenting part during delivery. Bladder tone and detrusor reflex may be diminished by trauma or anesthesia. Tears may extend into the urethra.

Resumption of urination requires relaxation and comfort, as well as a return of bladder tone. Early ambulation makes a bedpan largely unnecessary and helps to preclude problems of the woman trying to void from a horizontal position. Pelvic floor exercises prior to and after delivery help to restore bladder and urethral tone. A warm bedpan (if one has to be used), running water, and warm water over the vulva will help the woman to void. Voiding in the shower or sitz bath may be easier for the first time or two. Palpate the fundus and measure voiding, if possible, to assess emptying of the bladder.

Catheterization will be necessary if the woman is unable to void and her bladder is distended. It is not easy to catheterize a woman postpartum nor is it desirable to introduce an added risk of infection, so every effort and support should be directed toward helping the woman to void on her own. If, however, she is unable to void or to empty her bladder, an indwelling catheter may be placed for 24 to 36 or 48 hours to rest the bladder and allow it to heal, edema to subside, and bladder and urethral tone to return.

Diuresis is a normal postpartum occurrence and commences 24 to 48 hours after delivery. It is the body's attempt to return to equilibrium following pregnancy. Its occurrence should in no way inhibit fluid intake. Adequate fluids are necessary to prevent infection and constipation.

Weight Loss and Body Image

Dramatic weight loss occurs with delivery of the fetus, placenta, membranes, and amniotic fluid. Lochia, diminishing blood volume, and diuresis also contribute to weight loss. Initial postpartum weight loss does not continue, however, and women find that they are far from prepregnancy weight and shape after delivery. The woman's image of her body after delivery may resemble her prepregnant self (Rubin, 1984, pp. 122–124). Reality postpartum may be more pounds to lose, poor abdominal muscle tone, a sore perineum, leaking tender breasts, and persistent fat pads on buttocks, thighs, and abdomen, carryovers from pregnancy contours. There is often disruption of integrity of body functions. Urination is painful or even impossible, having a bowel movement is viewed as a major hurdle, lochia is profuse, and perineal pads are uncomfortable, especially to a woman socialized to use tampons. Her breasts may be sore and leak milk.

The woman may feel discomfort, or disfigurement, be weak or dizzy, have sore breasts, and feel a sense of trauma from the experience of labor and delivery (Carlson, 1976, p. 29). The woman may exhibit anxiety and a need for control. She may be very involved and almost obsessed with body functions: having a bowel movement, producing breast milk (Rubin, 1961, p. 75). Fawcett (1978) found that women demonstrated a decrease in perceived body space during the puerperium (p. 231). Women indicated that they "wanted to feel especially small early in the postpartum as a consequence of feeling so large and awkward in the later months of pregnancy" (p. 232).

Reva Rubin has stated that the postpartum period may be very cruel (1975, p. 1684). The woman needs a chance to recover before she is confronted with the many tasks parenting imposes. She needs time for what Rubin characterizes as the "taking-in phase." This is a time of regeneration and restoration, of need for deep sleep and food. The woman may exhibit passive dependent behavior (Rubin, 1961, p. 754). She may also exhibit behaviors of looking for approval (Rubin, 1961, p. 685). She needs relief from discomfort, but also to be reassured that the symptoms she has are normal (Fowler, 1971, p. 41).

The feelings a woman experiences postpartum are associated with her feelings about life and womanhood (Edwards, 1973/74, p. 19). Lack of support can contribute to physiologic processes of change and healing. If the woman is in conflict between her fantasy and real mother-role images, she may reflect this in the care she takes of herself (Edwards, 1973/74, p. 20). She needs time for adaptation to the tremendous hormonal changes that have taken place within her body (Jones, 1975, p. 52).

During the puerperium, the woman needs those closest to her, be it husband, friend, or significant other, to demonstrate that she is worthwhile, cared about, loved, and still physically attractive. If the repulsion she may feel about her own body with leaking breasts, lochia flow, wearing perineal pads which she may have discarded years before for tampons, and carrying extra pounds is reflected in those about her, her feelings of self-worth and her body image will be all the more negative. Imposed sexual abstinence may further deteriorate her image of herself as a woman. Pregnancy and the puerperium can be used to help the woman celebrate her womanhood and "the couple to develop and increase their sexual awareness, responsiveness, and intimacy with one another" (Kyndely, 1978, p. 32). It is important that we as caregivers not ignore the intimacy needs of couples during the postpartum hospital stay. They need time to be alone, to touch, hug, stroke, and to share intimacies in private. We need to be sensitive to allowing couples privacy and encouraging a variety of expressions of caring. Vaginal intercourse can be resumed when the woman is comfortable and the episiotomy (if present) has healed, but it should be considered only one means of expression of intimacy and caring. In Chapter 6, a section on teaching about sexuality after childbirth is included.

Developmental Tasks of the Puerperium

The woman is confronted with a number of important developmental tasks to be accomplished during the puerperium. She may expect a quick adaptation to a confusion of tasks and be dismayed when this does not occur (Carlson, 1976, p. 28). Biophysical tasks include involution of the reproductive organs, establishment of lactation or return of the breasts to a nonpregnant, nonlactating state, return to prepregnancy weight and body contours, restoration of muscle tone of the abdomen and pelvic soft tissues, and resumption of regular patterns of elimination. Initiation of these tasks should occur in the early days of the puerperium, beginning with the first assessment after delivery. Teaching about caretaking is one of the major roles of the maternity nurse and is discussed in detail in Chapter 6.

Psychosocial tasks include role realignment, acquisition of a new role, and integration of a new member into the family constellation. Components of the new role include those which are emotional and those concerned with caretaking. Parenthood implies new attitudes, beliefs, responsibilities, and relationships. Reorganization of both the household and the woman's identity must occur (Ludington-Hoe, 1977, p. 1171). The woman may resent the health and mobility of her husband, friends, significant others, and relatives. She may feel threatened by a fear of inadequacy, and advice from others may be perceived as criticism (Brown, 1975, p. 61).

Early assessment of the woman postpartum in relation to the developmental tasks, both biophysical and psychosocial, which she must accomplish will enable the nursing staff to utilize the time the woman spends in the postpartum unit for support and teaching and to make appropriate referrals for follow-up after discharge. Several tools have been developed to assist in the assessment process (Campbell & Smith, 1977, 1179; Sheehan, 1981, pp. 22–23). An example is included in Appendix B to guide in development of a tool appropriate to your particular institution and the population you serve.

Cultural Aspects of Care

Childbearing is a developmental event replete with cultural implications. It is impossible to separate this most important event, the creation and manifestation of a new life, from the traditions and beliefs each participant brings to the occasion. Therefore, it is imperative that we as caregivers familiarize ourselves with the cultures represented in our client populations.

Immigration of Arabs to the United States has accelerated in recent years. Most of these persons come from Lebanon, Palestine, Jordan, Syria, Iraq, Egypt, and countries along the Arabian Gulf (Meleis & Sorrell, 1981, p. 171). Since children are an integral part of all family events, separation from their mother during the birthing and postpartum experiences constitutes a break in tradition. Modesty of women is highly valued and must be respected by health care providers. Although sex and reproductive issues are freely discussed among Arab women, these issues are not discussed with men or strangers (Meleis & Sorrell, 1981, pp. 172–174).

Vietnamese refugees have been admitted to the United States in large numbers in the past few years. Thus, we as health care providers are working with a cultural group new to many of us. Vietnamese people view pregnancy as a normal, healthy process. Women expect to have their infants with them after birth, but also expect to have help with caretaking. It is difficult for Vietnamese women to discuss private health matters with others or to relegate care of the sick to anyone other than family (Grosso et al., 1981, pp. 177–179). Wadd found several important implications for postpartum nursing care in her study of Vietnamese women. She emphasizes inclusion of the family, translation of routine hospital diets into food acceptable to Vietnamese clients, offering the option of a basin of warm water to showering, and minimizing the drawing of blood samples on clients (a much feared procedure) (1983, p. 257).

Native American women may or may not retain their customs in relation to childbearing. It is especially important to realize that there are over 300 American Indian tribes in the United States, as well as Alaskan natives. Eliciting, accepting, and respecting values is most important in providing sensitive and humanistic care for women of Indian background (Farris, 1978, pp. 20–33).

Just as it is not possible to generalize about native Americans, so too is it impossible to do so for any other group which contributes to the melting pot of American heritage. Examples of traditions serve to illustrate the diversity of practices and, hopefully, so sensitize caregivers to understand and support practices which seem important to the women with whom they work. Black American women who often view pregnancy as a healthy normal event, may, to the contrary, view the puerperium as a "sick" time because of the presence of vaginal bleeding, and impose hygienic restrictions. Special foods may be given the woman and others avoided (Carrington, 1978, pp. 48–49).

Mexican American women may adhere to special practices including wearing an abdominal/perineal binder, dietary restrictions, bathing, and resumption of household duties (Kay, 1978, pp. 100–101).

Some Puerto Rican women fear that their husbands will go elsewhere if they look "awful" after delivery. Families who have immigrated to the mainland from Puerto Rico often lack support of extended families for childbearing tasks. Thus, these women are under particular stress to resume their household duties as soon as possible, as well as care for the infant and find time for rest to restore their own health (Sanavitis & Murillo-Rohde, 1978, pp. 119, 124).

These examples of traditions emphasize the importance not only of accepting our clients for who they are, but also discovering who they are (Spector, 1979, p. 293). Since most of us work primarily with only a few cultural groups, it should be possible to familiarize ourselves with practices surrounding the childbirth and puerperal experiences and adapt our caring to those practices. Members of target communities can be approached for assistance in sharing and clarifying beliefs, practices, taboos, and perceptions of developmental and situational events on the health–illness continuum, as well as understanding of the roles played by clients and providers. Health care can and should be a collaborative process with all the people whom we purport to serve. A sensitive and important time to build strong positive relationships that will have impact on the health of the whole family and the lifelong health of the new member is during the puerperium.

Summary

The woman's perceptual field is contracted at the end of pregnancy (Levine, 1976, p. 12).The puerperium represents a time for energy gathering and inner centering. The inner-directed field lowers the woman's ability to cope with her environment. She needs time to rest in order to regroup and cope with the tasks she must accomplish (Levine, 1976, pp. 12, 14).

The woman's perceptions of herself and the caretaking she receives will influence her abilities to cope with new tasks and roles and attain a high level of wellness. Knowledge of risk factors as a basis for assessment in the early puerperium can assist us as nurses to augment the woman's own coping strategies to assist her to remain in precrisis and be on her way toward achieving the biophysical and psychosocial tasks she must accomplish through the duration of the puerperium.

References

Brooten, D. A., Brown, L. P., Hollingsworth, A. O., Tanis, J. L., & Donlen, J. A comparison of four treatments to prevent and control breast pain and engorgement in nonnursing mothers. *Nursing Research*, 1983, *32*(4), 225–229.

Brown, C. Baby blues. *Nursing Mirror*, 1975, *141*(12), 61–62.

Campbell, S., & Smith, J. Postpartum: Assessment guide. *American Journal of Nursing*, 1977, *77*(7), 1179.

Carlson, S. E. The surreality of postpartum: Observations on the subjective experience. *Journal of Obstetric, Gynecologic and Neonatal Nursing*, 1976, *5*(5), 28.

Carrington, B. W. The Afro-American. In A. L. Clark (Ed.), *Culture childbearing health professionals*. Philadelphia: F. A. Davis, 1978, pp. 34–52.

Clark, A. L. *Culture childbearing health professionals*. Philadelphia: F. A. Davis, 1978.

Edwards, M. The crises of the fourth trimester. *Birth and Family Journal*, Winter 1973/74, *1*(1), 19–22.

Farris, L. The American Indian. In A. L. Clark (Ed.), *Culture childbearing health professionals.* Philadelphia: F. A. Davis, 1978, pp. 20–33.
Fawcett, J. Body image and the pregnant couple. *The American Journal of Maternal Child Nursing,* 1978, *3*(4), 227–233.
Fowler, M. M. Psychological need in the puerperium. In A. L. Clark (Ed.), *Maturational crisis of childbearing.* Honolulu: University of Hawaii, 1971, pp. 40–44.
Grosso, C., Barden, M., Henry, C., & Vieau, M. G. The Vietnamese American family . . . and grandma makes three. *The American Journal of Maternal Child Nursing,* 1981, *6*(3), 177–180.
Jones, W. L. The emotional needs of the new family. *Nursing Mirror,* 1975, *141*(17), 49–52.
Kay, M. A. The Mexican American. In A. L. Clark (Ed.), *Culture childbearing health professionals.* Philadelphia: F. A. Davis, 1978, pp. 88–108.
Kyndely, K. The sexuality of women in pregnancy and postpartum: A review. *Journal of Obstetric, Gynecologic and Neonatal Nursing,* 1978, *1*(1), 28–32.
Levine, N. H. A conceptual model for obstetric nursing. *Journal of Obstetric, Gynecologic and Neonatal Nursing,* 1976, *5*(2), 9–15.
Ludington-Hoe, S. M. Postpartum: Development of maternicity. *American Journal of Nursing,* 1977, *77*(7), 1171–1174.
Meleis, A. I., & Sorrell, L. Arab American women and their birth experiences. *The American Journal of Maternal Child Nursing,* 1981, *6*(3), 171–176.
Polden, M. Obstetric physiotherapy. *Nursing Mirror,* 1975, *141*(1), 54–57.
Rising, S. The fourth stage of labor: Family integration. *American Journal of Nursing,* 1974, *74*(5), 870–874.
Rubin, R. Basic maternal behavior. *Nursing Outlook,* 1961, *9*(11), 683–686.
Rubin, R. Puerperal change. *Nursing Outlook,* 1961, *9*(12), 753–755.
Rubin, R. Maternity nursing stops too soon. *American Journal of Nursing,* 1975, *75*(10), 1680–1684.
Rubin, R. *Maternal identity and the maternal experience.* New York: Springer Publishing Company, 1984.
Sanavitis, A. M., & Murillo-Rohde, I. The Puerto Rican. In A. L. Clark (Ed.), *Culture childbearing health professionals.* Philadelphia: F. A. Davis, 1978, pp. 110–126.
Sheehan, F. Assessing postpartum adjustment. *Journal of Obstetric, Gynecologic and Neonatal Nursing,* 1981, *10*(1), 19–23.
Spector, R. E. *Cultural diversity in health and illness.* New York: Appleton-Century-Crofts, 1979.
Thompson, M. A. *Shock syndrome.* Menlo Park, Calif.: Addison-Wesley, 1978.
Wadd, L. Vietnamese postpartum practices. *Journal of Obstetric, Gynecologic and Neonatal Nursing,* 1983, *12*(4), 252–258.

4

Risks During the Puerperium for the Woman

Introduction

The postpartum unit is, in general, a happy place. Since childbirth is a normal developmental event for most women and their families, the puerperium marks a beginning and a transition. It is a time of restoration, of change, of growth for the woman, her infant, and perhaps the child's father, significant others, friends, and family. Most women and their infants remain in precrisis as they meet the challenges to reproductive integrity successfully.

For some women and/or their infants, however, the insult to integrity, biophysical and/or psychosocial, exceeds coping abilities. Unless external resources are successful in augmenting the individual's or family's attempts to remain in precrisis, crisis will occur.

Working with childbearing families who are experiencing crisis can be threatening to nurses who work in the maternity setting, since clients may be similar in age to staff members. Facing crises is inconsistent with their work patterns and routine on the postpartum unit. "Death or serious compromise in health seems especially difficult to confront in the young" (Hawkins & Higgins, 1981, p. 427). Since both clients and providers expect a positive outcome from the birthing and postpartum experience, it is all the more important that support and caring be extended to women and their families when crises occur.

In a small book entitled *Marriage and Motherhood,* Davidson emphasizes the fact that pregnancy and labor are natural conditions and goes on to say, "it must be remembered that though this is so they set up a state in the woman which is on the borderland of disease, and the boundary line is easily passed, so that all possible precautions should be taken to keep the mother well and healthy" (undated, pp. 66–67).

Nurses are the prime caretakers who can meet the challenge that this statement implies through their knowledge and expertise in care of women and their infants during the critical first days of the puerperium.

In this chapter, we will explore risks that can exist for the woman during the puerperium. Those risks related to parenting and the infant will be addressed in Chapter 7.

Assessment for Risk Factors

Recognition of the potential for crisis is an important factor in helping women to remain in precrisis throughout the duration of the puerperium. Identification of those women at particular risk for selected situational hazardous events such as hemorrhage, infection, toxemia, or depression constitutes primary prevention for the puerperium. Both biophysical and psychosocial crises can occur as a direct result of the birth experience or precipitated by events upon which pregnancy is superimposed. A thorough past health history and use of the Holmes/Rahe Social Readjustment Scale (see Appendix C) as well as knowledge of development stages, are useful in predicting the potential for crisis and planning management strategies to augment the coping of the individual and/or family to avert crisis. Risk factors common to women during the puerperium are listed in Table 4.1. These will be discussed from the perspective of nursing augmentation and interventions in this chapter and in Chapter 7.

Loss of Reproductive Integrity

The woman who has just delivered is subject to a number of risks related directly to her reproductive organs and their repair and involution to a nonpregnant state. Most of these are a direct result of the labor and delivery experience. Establishment of lactation, however, is not directly related, and the decision to have a tubal ligation is, of course, an elective means to terminate fertility.

Hemorrhage. Excessive bleeding during the puerperium is defined by some authors as loss of over 500 milliliters, but other references use the figure of 1,000 milliliters. Hemorrhage remains the second leading cause of maternal death in this country (Easterling, 1977, p. 719).

Table 4.1 Risk Factors Common to Women During the Puerperium

Risk Category	Selected Hazardous Events
Loss of Reproductive Integrity	failure to establish lactation uterine atony tubal ligation lacerations episiotomy Caesarean section removal of reproductive organs
Loss of Relationships	disruption/failure in attachment processes with infant "blues" puerperal depression puerperal psychosis divorce disinterest/disappearance of significant other interruption of career, job
Loss of Patency	urinary retention constipation thrombophlebitis disseminated intravascular coagulation pulmonary embolus
Loss of Regulation	toxemia diabetes
Loss of Protective Mechanisms	puerperal sepsis cystitis mastitis
Loss of Mobility	thrombophlebitis Caesarean section

The most common cause of hemorrhage during the puerperium is uterine atony. Factors that put the woman at greater risk for hemorrhage due to uterine atony are as follows: overdistention of the uterus for a number of reasons including polyhydramnios; multiple gestation; a large fetus; grandmultiparity; prolonged labor; excessive or inappropriate use of oxytocins; relaxation of uterine muscle secondary to use of general anesthesia; retention of secundae; undetected or prolonged urinary retention; and overvigorous massage of the uterus following delivery. The first course of action, when uterine atony is detected, is to massage the fundus gently. If the uterus is at or above the level of the umbilicus, displaced to the right, and atonic, the bladder should be palpated and every effort made to have the woman void. Catheterization may be necessary if bladder sensation is absent in order to empty the bladder to allow the uterus to involute normally. Unless evidence points to overzealous use of oxytocins as a cause of atony, oxytocins by intravenous, intramuscular, or oral route are used to promote involution. Breast-feeding stimulates oxytocin release and is one measure that may be used to combat atony. Failure of the uterus to contract with cautious and judicious use of any or all the above measures with continued atony and bright red bleeding suggests retention of placental fragments and/or membranes, necessitating more vigorous medical intervention. It should be noted that this is also a major cause of hemorrhage after the first 24 hours. A curettage is done to remove retained secundae. Rarely, ligation of the hypogastric arteries or hysterectomy are done if bleeding is continuous, less extreme interventions fail, and the woman's life is threatened.

In the absence of uterine atony, excessive bright red bleeding suggests lacerations of cervix, vagina, and/or perineum. Prompt inspection and repair are necessary to prevent continued blood loss. Nursing assessment is critical to early detection of excess bleeding and its cause.

Hematomas usually occur in the area of the episiotomy and are often visible or apparent through clinical signs of blood loss in the absence of excessive lochia and uterine atony and swelling and pain in the perineum. Rarely, a hematoma may occur in the broad ligament through rupture of a deep vessel (Easterling, 1977, p. 719). In either case, evacuation and ligation of vessels may be necessary. Occasionally, hysterectomy is the only choice.

Causes of hemorrhage that are less common are placenta accreta and rupture of the uterus. The former is usually apparent during the third stage of labor and the latter is usually a phenomenon of labor rather than of the puerperium.

Episiotomy. Episiotomies are often done routinely, especially on primigravidous women, to provide adequate room for birth of the head and prevent uncontrolled lacerations. It is argued that a clean episiotomy incision is easier to repair than a jagged tear which may extend through the anal mucosa (fourth-degree laceration). Midline episiotomy is usually the procedure of choice. This episiotomy, when properly repaired, heals quickly and is the least painful. A mediolateral episiotomy is more painful and takes longer to heal.

For the woman who was unprepared for the pain of an episiotomy, this event may represent crisis. If a mediolateral was performed or if complications such as extension of a median into the anal muscle or through the mucosa or a hematoma occur, the woman may be uncomfortable, unable to sit to feed her infant, and afraid to evacuate her bowels. An unexpected episiotomy may be a symbol of failure for the woman or of loss of control. It is often easy for us as providers to accept episiotomies as routine and forget that the woman's perception of the event may be far from routine.

Removal of reproductive organs. When hysterectomy is necessary secondary to events surrounding the birth experience, the woman is subjected not only to the biophysical stresses of major surgery, but also to the psychosocial aspects of loss of reproductive integrity. Grieving reactions are common. The woman may experience feelings of loss of her femininity (Humphries, 1980, p. 2). Since the hysterectomy would occur as a result of biophysical crisis, rather than as a planned event in response to unabating symptoms over time, the woman would have no time to rally her coping mechanisms. There is little time, too, for preparation of the woman for the procedure, her expected postoperative course, and the effects it will have on her life.

Reactions to hysterectomy are those common to stages of the grieving process. Women at particular risk for depression are those younger than 40 (thus, in their childbearing years) (Richards, 1973, pp. 430–432). Other women at risk are those who characterize themselves as "half a woman" or "empty" and those whose significant others use words such as "desexed," "neuter," or "a shell of a woman" (Melody, 1962, pp. 410–413).

Faced with the expected role alterations in relation to parenthood, and possible disruption of her career due to the prolonged recovery time required after major surgery, the woman who has had a hysterectomy postpartum needs special support to remain in precrisis with regard to her identity, body image, and role functioning. In addition, nursing interventions must be aimed at postcrisis restoration and return to a higher level of wellness following the biophysical assault and crisis which resulted in hysterectomy.

It is obvious from the literature that many women have fears about and believe in myths surrounding loss of the uterus (Cosper, Fuller, & Robinson, 1978, p. 7). For women still in their childbearing years and perhaps desiring more children, the procedure may be even more dreaded. Hysterectomy may represent the end to reproduction before it is desired, with the attendant risk of precipitating crisis for the woman in terms of her identity and role functioning as a sexual being.

Recovery postpartum will be more complex for the woman who has had a hysterectomy. Since a hysterectomy following childbirth is seldom a planned event, opportunity for preoperative teaching will be minimal. Postoperative teaching, care, and preparation for discharge become even more important to the woman's achievement of a higher level of wellness postcrisis. Assessments will include urinary character and output, abdominal and perineal dressings and pads, and vital signs (Hawkins & Higgins, 1981, p. 485). The incision line should be observed for healing and for signs of infection. Early ambulation is encouraged to prevent flatus, emboli, and lung problems, as well as promoting circulation, restoration of normal patterns of elimination, and feelings of well-being. Prior to ambulation, regular turning, coughing, and deep breathing help to prevent stasis of respiratory secretions and formation of thrombi.

Expected biophysical alterations following hysterectomy are both temporary and permanent. Temporary alterations include restrictions in lifting of heavy objects and in performing heavy work such as vacuuming or house cleaning for a month or more. The woman can expect to feel tired more often for several weeks and should, therefore, pace household tasks, infant care, and social activities. Restrictions on driving and resumption of vaginal intercourse may be recommended for four to six weeks. Spotting is normal about two weeks after the procedure when internal sutures are absorbed, but bright red vaginal bleeding and/or foul-smelling discharge are signs of complications.

If the adnexa have been removed as well as the uterus, the woman will experience abrupt onset of menopausal symptoms. Menstruation will, of course, occur no more. If the ovaries are still in place, they will continue to function until the time of menopause. Sexual functioning should be minimally affected if the ovaries are intact (Finck, 1979, p. 292). The woman's body image will, of course, be altered due to the presence of an abdominal scar. She needs information about healing of the incision and the eventual appearance of the scar.

Discharge planning is more complex for the woman who has had a new baby and a hysterectomy concurrently. Realistic plans for discharge include identification and mobilization of internal and external resources. Some examples appear in Table 4.2. Family members and/or significant others should be included in planning, so they as well as the woman are aware of the limitations on her activity and projected time for recovery.

In one study, women (13–100%) reported disruptions in the following activities five weeks posthysterectomy: sleeping, eating, bowel movements, voiding, energy level, household work, and leisure pursuits (Cosper et al., 1978, pp. 7–11).

Tubal ligation. Tubal ligation, although an elective procedure, re-

Table 4.2 Resources

Internal	External
nutritional status	family
general state of health	friends
genetics	significant others
	visiting nurse services
	financial insurance Medicaid membership in prepaid plan
	clergy
	home health care services
	babysitters
	day care; nursery school
	nurses and other health care providers in hospital and community
	education
	environment home community

quires a decision on the part of the woman, and perhaps her husband or significant other, as well, to end the childbearing function of her (their) sexuality. Reasons for choosing sterilization are important to explore prior to the time of the procedure. Misinformation about reversibility may lead the woman to believe it is a method used to delay having children. Sterilization is not a panacea for marriage problems, financial worries, or sexual hang-ups. A realistic assessment of possible future circumstances should help the woman to decide whether or not she is willing to accept an end to her fertility (Planned Parenthood, 1978, p. 3). The woman should also be prepared for the biophysical aspects of the procedure. The procedure may be done through a small abdominal incision whereby the tubes are either clamped or cut and the ends sutured, or a fimbriectomy (amputation of the fimbrial ends of the tubes) can be performed. These procedures may also be done transvaginally through an incision in the cul-de-sac, but would rarely if every be done by this route postpartally. The laparoscopic technique involves a tiny incision in the umbilical area and a second tiny incision in the right or left lower quadrant. The tubes are visualized with the laparoscope and then cauterized. Newer techniques eliminate electrocautery and make use of silicone bands or spring-loaded clips to occlude the tubes.

Tubal ligation in the immediate postpartum period may prolong hospitalization by a day or so. With the abdominal procedure, the woman should be prepared for recovery similar to that of any simple abdominal surgery procedure. Laparoscopic techniques have the lowest rates of complication and a shorter recovery period. Referred shoulder pain sometimes occurs in the first day or two after the procedure, probably because of irritation of the diaphragm from air in the peritoneal cavity.

Cesarean section. The woman who has had a cesarean section has not only had a baby, but has also undergone a major surgical procedure. A C-section also means a temporary loss or threat to mobility. Her biophysical recovery may be complicated by her feelings about having a section and the reasons for the choice of this route for delivery. Preparation for a planned cesarean can be far more leisurely and comprehensive than when the section is done under crisis conditions.

All of the care common to clients who have undergone abdominal surgery is applicable for women who have had sections. Evaluation of biophysical status progresses from quarter hourly vital signs and assessment of lochia flow to hourly, every four hours, four times a day, and even daily assessments, depending upon the woman's recovery and institutional protocols. Leg exercises, turning, coughing and deep breathing, and early ambulation will help to prevent complications of respiratory and circulatory stasis.

The woman may have an intravenous line for the first few hours or day. Once normal bowel sounds resume and nausea subsides, progressive oral feedings begin.

Assessment of bleeding, both vaginal and incisional, is frequent at first. Due to the abdominal incision and possible presence of skin clips, sutures, staples, and/or a dressing and abdominal binder, it is difficult to palpate the fundus. Lochia flow must be evaluated through pad counts and vital signs.

An indwelling urinary catheter may be in place for the first 24 to 36 or 48 hours or may be removed as early as in the recovery room. Signs and symptoms of urinary retention and infection are important to recognize. Pelvic floor exercises are helpful to restore bladder and uretheral tone.

Relief of pain is important to the woman's recovery and sense of well-being. Use of analgesics and other pain relief measures such as backrubs, a well placed binder, and ambulation should be evaluated for efficacy. Warm showers are very soothing and are often permitted three to four days postoperatively. Skin clips or staples are removed six to seven days after surgery.

The meaning of cesarean section to the woman should not be ignored. Cox and Smith (1982) found in their study that women who have had a cesarean section had lower self-esteem than those women who had delivered vaginally (p. 313). Postpartum, this woman may need support in coping with a perceived loss of reproductive integrity and of her feelings of failure as a woman for being unable to deliver vaginally. She may need information about the procedure, the reasons for it, and what she can expect for future pregnancies. The meaning of a cesarean to the woman in the context of her cultural group should be recognized and explored. The woman may feel a sense of loss of control over her body, magnified by having her baby ''taken'' from her and the presence of an incision.

Assumption of responsibility for infant care will be delayed. Inclusion of the child's father, if he is interested and willing, will help the couple work together in learning to care for their child (Harris, 1980, p. 202).

Loss of Relationships

The woman may be faced with losses or disruptions in her relationships with others following the birth of her child. The attachment process with her infant may be disrupted if she has had a cesarean and/or if the child experiences a crisis in adaptation to extrauterine life and needs special care. Women who are undergoing life changes such as divorce, loss of a significant other, or death of a loved one are faced with the tasks of attachment with their children at the same time they are experiencing loss. The woman for whom pregnancy and birth mean interruption of a career also experience loss of the relationships inherent in the job. All of these will be addressed in Chapters 5, 6, and 7.

The ''blues,'' puerperal depression, and psychosis are phenomena unique to the childbirth experience. They may occur immediately or several weeks or months after delivery. Most women experience only transient ''blues,'' a period of labile emotions and mild depression. As many as 80 percent of women experience postpartum ''blues'' somewhere between 2 and 10 days after delivery. "Blues" are characterized by periods of despondency, fatigue, tearfulness, anxiety, and poor concentration (Hatrick, 1976, pp. 533–534). They are probably due to the dramatic fall in estrogens and progesterones and the dramatic changes in blood chemistry which result when the placenta is delivered (Ritchie, 1977, pp. 14–17).

The puerperium represents a time of dramatic role changes, family disruption, and demands on the woman. Biophysical as well as psychosocial adaptations are necessary to avert crisis. Women report feeling isolated, tied down, and experiencing emotional tension after delivery (Gruis, 1977). Melchior reports that women commonly experience feelings of depression, loneliness, and fatigue during the puerperium (1975, pp. 30–32). For most women, however, with care, sensitivity, and support of health professionals, family, and/or significant others, the "blues" will be self-limiting, transient, and minimally disruptive.

Postpartum depression occurs much less frequently, affecting some 10 percent of women (Black, 1975, p. 266). Other figures cited are 3 to 23 percent (Ritchie, 1977, p. 14). There is a range of intensity in symptoms experienced, but women generally experience a persistent mood change and at least some disruption of normal events (Cogan, 1980, p. 1). Frequent complaints of women include sleep disturbances, decreased appetite, loss of libido, increased fatigue, constipation, and weight loss (Ritchie, 1977, p. 15). Since all of these can occur postpartum, diagnosis of depression is based on degree and extent of symptoms as well as their occurrence. The woman may report feeling sad, depressed, or blue, have crying spells, and experience loss of emotional attachments. Feelings of hopelessness, low self-esteem, self-criticism, lack of motivation, distortion of body image, inability to cope with the infant, and increased dependency may occur. Suicidal wishes and avoidance wishes may also occur. Objective data relate to appearance: speech, dress, hygiene, weight, facies, eye contact, and posture. Activity may reflect regression or agitation (Ritchie, 1977, pp. 15–16). Causes of depression include changes in blood chemistry and the abrupt changes parenthood implies. Postpartum depression has been linked with maternal age (22 to 30 years) and inversely with the degree of assistance, love, and support received from the husband (Frate et al., 1979, p. 363). It has also been linked with societal expectations (Tentoni & High, 1980, p. 248).

Interventions during pregnancy with women identified as at risk have been demonstrated to make a difference in the occurrence of depression (Forecasting, 1980, p. 119). Postpartum depression has the potential for being long-term, so early treatment is a must (Pitt, 1968, pp. 1325–1335). One woman who experienced depression suggests that women need to care for their infants as much as they are able. She stresses the need to listen; that even depressed women know what they need. Sometimes the husband, who has looked forward to birth, and is experiencing joy and pride, is not the best person to help. Professional health care providers can support and help both partners (Thomas, 1979, p. 34). It is also important to support women, particularly primiparas, in coping with societal attitudes toward pregnancy which adversely affect self-image and self-esteem (Tentoni & High, 1980, p. 248). Men, too, need support as they have been shown to suffer depression postpartum: crying, sensitivity, and general blues (*Ms.*, 1981, p. 18). Bieber and Bieber report instances in which men experienced reactions postpartum, including tearfulness (1978, pp. 511–519).

Puerperal psychoses are the least frequent in occurrence and the most severe. The rate is about four cases per thousand women (Kendell et al., 1976, pp. 297–302). Psychoses account for 2 to 8 percent of admissions to mental hospitals (Herzog & Detre, 1976, p. 229). Most episodes occur within two weeks of delivery. An interesting but inconclusive link between severity of affective disturbances and free plasma tryptophan levels has been demonstrated. Queries have also been raised as to a relationship with estrogen and progesterone secretion (Stein et al., 1976, p. 457). Clinical features include clouding of consciousness, incoherence, sleep disturbances, nightmares, and depressive episodes (Hatrick, 1976, p. 533). The woman may experience profound disruption in behavior. She may have hallucinations or delusions (Woollaston, 1973, p. 145).

Treatment may include institutionalization or outpatient therapy. Several authors urge that the woman and her infant not be separated if at all possible (Hatrick, 1976; Woollaston, 1973). Support, help in setting priorities, plenty of sleep, assistance with child care and/or household tasks, and a good diet may all be beneficial. Parent discussion groups can be supportive to role transitions necessitated by birth (Hawkins & Higgins, 1981, p. 435).

Loss of Patency

Urinary retention and constipation represent minor, nonthreatening risks to the woman during the puerperium. They will be discussed under self-care in Chapter 6. Thrombophlebitis, amniotic fluid embolus, disseminated intravascular coagulation, and pulmonary embolus are life-threatening, although rare, examples of crises women may experience. They represent loss of patency in the circulatory system and are not unique to the puerperium. They are, however, sufficiently common during this time to warrant discussion.

Thrombophlebitis. Although this occurs in fewer than one percent of all women during the puerperium, it occurs more frequently than in nonpregnant women (Easterling, 1977, p. 718). Early ambulation as well as generally better health and fewer traumatic deliveries have led to a decrease in incidence. This condition was known as "white leg" and onset was described as occurring between 5 and 21 days postpartum (Davidson, undated, p. 64). This was at a time when women were generally kept in bed for three weeks.

The cause of deep vein thrombosis has been attributed to trauma to pelvic veins from pressure of the presenting part, sluggish circulation in large venous sinuses, and alterations in coagulation related to the large amounts of estrogens produced during pregnancy. Estrogen-containing drugs once commonly in use to suppress lactation have also been implicated.

Classical signs include pain and tenderness, fever, a positive Homan's, and usually increased circumference of the affected part. Doppler ultrasound or venography can be used to confirm the diagnosis. Endoparametritis and pelvic cellulitis which do not respond to antibiotics should be cause for suspicion of pelvic thrombophlebitis.

Bed rest, elevation of the affected extremity, analgesics, and elastic stockings are usually sufficient for superficial venous thrombosis (Easterling, 1977, p. 718). For deep vein thrombosis, use of anticoagulants may be necessary along with bed rest and physical therapy. This crisis also represents loss of mobility and a threat to the woman's ability to care for herself and her infant.

Pulmonary embolus. Occasionally, in spite of rigorous intervention, pulmonary embolism occurs. The woman may experience shortness of breath, chest pain, a cough and possible hemoptysis, fever, and tachycardia. Auscultation reveals a friction rub and signs of plural effusion and possible atelectasis. Anticoagulants are the therapy of choice, along with supportive measures to maintain respiratory integrity. If emboli recur, ligation of the vena cava and ovarian veins may be contemplated (Easterling, 1977, p. 718). The biophysical crisis this disorder represents not only disrupts return to health, but also can precipitate a psychosocial crisis for the woman. Caught in the demands role changes impose, she needs care and support to focus her energies on weathering the crisis of the body insult. Contact with her infant will be important to attachment and her feelings of self-worth as a woman. She needs reassurance that she will, in time, be able to assume more care of her baby and herself.

Disseminated intravascular coagulation. DIC results from the stimultaneous action of thrombin and the fibrinolytic system. It can be triggered by retention of a dead fetus, saline infusion, amniotic fluid embolus, abruptio placenta, and septic shock (Conklin, 1974, p. 30). The substances triggering all of this may come from the placenta, serum from a retroplacental clot, from the amniotic fluid contaminated by catabolic products of fetolysis (as in retention of a dead fetus), or from amniotic debris as in a fluid embolism (Hasson, 1974, p. 28). Thrombin (a proteolytic enzyme) actions result in formation of fibrin. Specific clotting factors are consumed and there is aggregation and loss of platelets. The fibrinolytic system is also activated. The client presents with symptoms of diffuse hemorrhage and fibrin thrombus formation (Franco, 1979, p. 22). Hemorrhagic features of DIC occur because of the fibrinolysis that occurs (Franco, 1979, p. 25).

Hemorrhage is usually generalized and the woman may have petechiae, purpura, and extensive ecchymoses. There may be signs of gastrointestinal or genitourinary bleeding, as well as vaginal (Bell, 1977, p. 185). Thrombosis is exaggerated in the puerperium when both blood fibrinogen content and the platelet count are elevated and platelets are more sticky. Estrogens once widely used to suppress lactation increase risk (Cooper, 1976, p. 65).

Management is aimed at treatment of the resulting hypovolemia, use of heparin to disseminate thrombi, removal of the source of the problem, and careful monitoring of circulatory and renal function (Hasson, 1974, p. 28).

Supporting the woman and her family through this life-threatening crisis involves both monitoring of responses to medical interventions and nursing interventions aimed at supplementing the woman's own resources (O'Brian & Woods, 1978, p. 1880). Additionally, the woman who has looked forward to caring for and perhaps breast-feeding her child is now confronted with disruption of these important activities. She and her family need to understand what has happened and why. If the infant is stillborn or has died, she needs help to begin the grieving process. In Chapter 7, a complete discussion of loss and grieving is included.

Loss of Regulation

Toxemia. Rarely, toxemia occurs in the puerperium, usually within the first 48 hours. Reports of cases occurring as late as eleven days after delivery have been recorded in the literature, however.

Seizures in the absence of previous history or high fever occurring during the puerperium should be viewed as possibly the result of late toxemia (Late-date eclampsia, 1980, p. 109).

The woman who appears nervous and exhibits self-conscious movements, breathlessness, lack of confidence, trembling hands, and intolerance of noise should be followed closely for signs of impending eclampsia (Low, 1975, p. 1671). Blood pressure should be assessed based not only on pregnancy readings, but also on the prepregnancy baseline data. Onset of puerperal diuresis, urinary output, weight loss, reflexes, and any edema should be carefully observed and recorded. If the woman has seized during pregnancy, labor, and delivery, magnesium sulfate may be continued 24 to 48 hours after delivery (Wheeler & Jones, 1981, p. 223). However, women have been known to suffer eclamptic convulsions postpartum with no history during pregnancy. Therefore, all women should be carefully monitored postpartum for signs of toxemia.

A rare complication of eclampsia postpartum is intracerebral hemorrhage. Among those women who die secondary to eclampsia, however, the rate of this complication is 10 to 60 percent. If a woman is eclamptic and develops abnormal levels of consciousness or focal neurological signs, intracerebral hemorrhage should be suspected (Beck & Menezes, 1981).

Diabetes. The woman with diabetes upon which a pregnancy has been superimposed needs special care during the puerperium. Delivery of the placenta means removal of an insulin antagonist and signals return to a nonpregnant hormonal state. Women with diabetes are especially susceptible to toxemia, and this risk extends into the puerperium. Hemorrhage is an important risk because of uterine atony. Infants of diabetic women are often macrosomic, and hydramnios is a common occurrence. The risk of infections is greater. Adjustment of diet and insulin requirements to the nonpregnant state must occur during the puerperium to avoid insulin shock and coma (Rancilio, 1979, p. 453). Maintenance of normal blood glucose levels requires regular monitoring, adjustment of insulin, and accommodation of the catabolic activity of the puerperium (Rancilio, 1979, p. 454). Glucose tolerance improves dramatically after delivery and required insulin doses may drop one-fourth to one-half (Moore, Bingham, & Keesling, 1981, p. 193). The woman with gestational diabetes needs to understand the risks of developing diabetes and preventive measures with diet and weight control to preserve pancreatic function (Moore et al., 1981, p. 193).

Support, information and education for self-care and infant care, and preparation for discharge are important elements of care.

Loss of Protective Mechanisms

Sepsis during the puerperium is an important risk and one that is often treated lightly by health care providers because of the availability of antibiotics. It should be noted that infection is still one of the three leading causes of maternal mortality and morbidity, along with hemorrhage and toxemia.

The original definition of puerperal morbidity by the U.S. Joint Committee on Maternal Welfare states that it is a temperature of 100.4°F (38.0°C) in any 2 of the first 10 days postpartum excluding the first 24 hours, with the temperature being taken at least four times a day. Now with early discharge and early use of and response to antibiotics, this definition is quick to be dispelled. Some authorities now regard as morbid a temperature greater than 99.4°F or greater than 101°F after the second day, accompanied by clinical signs and symptoms of infection and a positive culture (Gibbs & Weinstein, 1976, p. 769).

Low-grade temperatures are very common in the early postpartum period and are related to dehydration, response to fetal proteins, genital or urinary tract infections, mastitis, breast abcesses, and upper respiratory infections. Predisposing factors include cesarean section, prolonged rupture of membranes, traumatic delivery, anemia, and low socioeconomic status. Other factors include vaginal examinations during labor, manual removal of the placenta, episiotomy, forceps delivery, and internal monitoring (Gibbs & Weinstein, 1976, pp. 770–773).

Infections are sometimes difficult to diagnose as to cause because many organisms may be normal inhabitants of the vagina and cervix. Most common causative organisms include: *Escherichia coli*, anaerobic streptococci, *Clostridium perfingens* (endogenous in up to 10 percent of women), gram negative aerobic bacilli, enterococcus, *Proteus, Klebsiella, Pseudomonas, Staphlococcus,* alpha and beta streptococcus, pneumococcus, *Listeria*, candida, and gonococcus (Gibbs & Weinstein, 1976, p. 779; Schwarz & Fruiterman, 1976, pp. 561–562).

Clinical signs and symptoms vary with the site of the infection. Infections of the genital tract present with diffuse and nonspecific symptoms: malaise, fever, and anorexia. Perineal and/or perirectal pain are later symptoms. Thrombophlebitis of pelvic veins with deep vein tenderness may also occur.

The endometrium is the most common site for puerperal infection. Known at one time as childbed fever, it was transmitted from woman to woman on the hands of providers. Semmelweis, an Austrian physician, recognized the mode of transmission in the early nineteenth century, but was discredited by colleagues (Thompson, 1949). Pain and foul-smelling lochia are classical signs.

Parametritis involves the broad ligament, but may also include the tubes, ovaries, and pelvic peritoneum (Easterling, 1977, p. 716). Generalized peritonitis may also occur, usually secondary to endoparametritis resulting from surgical delivery. Perineal infections are usually limited to the episiotomy or site of a laceration, often associated with small hematomas. Pain is the classic symptom, with swelling of the affected area.

Urinary tract infections must be differentiated from pelvic involvement. Classic signs of cystitis are usually present: pain and/or burning on urination, frequency, urgency, and sometimes hematuria. Trauma from birth and resultant need for catheterization are the usual precipitating events.

Mastitis is rarely seen in the hospital now that early discharges are common. Caused most commonly by *Staphylococcus aureus,* the route of infection may be a fissure in the nipple or not apparent. The parenchyma, ducts, and glands are usually involved. Pain, erythema, and induration make the presence and site of infection obvious (Easterling, 1977, p. 717).

Medical interventions for each of the infections described revolve around use of an antibiotic to which the organism is sensitive. Since most cases of cystitis are caused by *E. coli,* sulfonamides may be the drugs of choice. Adequate fluids, analgesics and pain-relief measures, good diet, and rest are important. Local application of heat may provide pain relief with mastitis and perineal infections. Curettage is a must if endometritis is related to retained secundae. In rare instances of endoparametritis, the infected organs must be removed. Special risks to women with infections include septic shock, renal failure, and DIC (Gibbs & Weinstein, 1976, p. 780).

Nursing interventions focus on providing external resources: adequate fluids, a diet supportive of healing processes, prescribed drugs, and appropriate comfort measures. The woman may be separated from her infant and needs support for coping with separation. Mastitis may temporarily disrupt or make breast-feeding uncomfortable. The woman needs support and caring to continue if that is her desire and there are no contraindications.

Summary

The woman who experiences crisis during the puerperium needs special caring from health care providers in order to weather the crisis and move to a higher level of wellness postcrisis. Interventions must focus not only on the biophysical aspects of crisis, if such occur, but also on the psychosocial. The tasks confronting the woman as she copes with role changes, biophysical adaptation, and the acquaintance process with her infant are awesome. A puerperal crisis may disrupt attachment, delay biophysical adaptation to a nonpregnant state, and/or affect role adaptation. Sensitivity to developmental events as well as attention to the crisis evolve from a holistic approach to care. Not to be forgotten, too, are the infant, other family members, friends, and significant others. Each will be affected by and have his or her own perceptions of the crisis. The caring aspects and holistic perspective we as nurses bring to the postpartum woman and those important to her can be critical in helping her achieve growth through crisis resolution.

References

Beck, D. W., & Menezes, A. H. Intracerebral hemorrhage in a patient with eclampsia. *Journal of the American Medical Association*, 1981, *246*(13), 1442–1443.

Bell, W. R. Hematologic abnormalities in pregnancy. *Medical Clinics of North America*, 1977, *61*(1), 165–199.

Bieber, I., & Bieber, T. B. Postpartum reactions in men and women. *Journal of the American Academy of Psychoanalysis*, 1978, *6*, 511–519.

Black, D. Pain and parenting. *Midwife and Health Visitor*, 1975, *11*(8), 263–266.

Cogan, R. Postpartum depression. *ICEA Review*, 1980, *4*(2), 1.

Conklin, M. M. DIC in the pregnant patient. *Journal of Obstetric, Gynecologic and Neonatal Nursing*, 1974, *3*(3), 29–32.

Cooper, K. Thrombosis and embolism in obstetrics. *Nursing Mirror*, 1976, *142*(11), 65–67.

Cosper, B., Fuller, S. S., & Robinson, G. J. Characteristics of post-hospitalization recovery following hysterectomy. *Journal of Obstetric, Gynecologic and Neonatal Nursing*, 1978, *7*(3), 7–11.

Cox, B. E., & Smith, E. C. The mother's self-esteem after a cesarean delivery. *The American Journal of Maternal Child Nursing*, 1982, *7*(5), 309–314.

Davidson, H. S. *Marriage and motherhood.* London: T. C. & E. C. Jack, undated.

Easterling, W. E. The puerperium. In D. N. Danforth (Ed.), *Obstetrics and gynecology* (3rd ed.). New York: Harper & Row, 1977, pp. 708–721.

Finck, K. S. The potential health care crisis of hysterectomy. In D. K. Kjervik & I. M. Martinson, *Women in stress: A nursing perspective.* New York: Appleton-Century-Crofts, 1979, pp. 276–302.

Forecasting the afterbirth. *Emergency Medicine*, 1980, *12*, 118–119.

Franco, L. M. Acute disseminated intravascular coagulation. *Cardiovascular Nursing*, 1979, *15*(5), 22–27.

Frate, D. A., Cowen, J. B., Rutledge, A. H., & Glasser, M. Behavioral reactions during the postpartum period: Experiences of 108 women. *Women & Health*, 1979, *4*(4), 355–371.

Gibbs, S., & Weinstein, A. J. Puerperal infection in the antibiotic era. *American Journal of Obstetrics and Gynecology*, 1976, *124*(7), 769–787.
Gruis, M. Beyond maternity: Postpartum concerns of mothers. *The American Journal of Maternal Child Nursing*, 1977, *2*(3), 182–188.
Harris, J. K. Self-care is possible after Cesarean delivery. *Nursing Clinics of North America*, 1980, *15*(1), 191–204.
Hasson, H. M. The role of enzymes in disseminated intravascular coagulation: An overview. *Journal of Obstetric, Gynecologic and Neonatal Nursing*, 1974, *3*(3), 27–29.
Hatrick, J. A. Puerperal mental illness. *Nursing Times*, 1976, *72*(14), 533–534.
Hawkins, J. W., & Higgins, L. P. *Maternity and gynecological nursing women's health care*. Philadelphia: J. B. Lippincott, 1981.
Herzog, A., & Detre, T. Psychotic reactions associated with childbirth. *Diseases of the Nervous System*, 1976, *37*(4), 229–235.
Humphries, P. T. Sexual adjustment after a hysterectomy. *Issues in Health Care of Women*, 1980, *2*(2), 1–14.
Kendell, R. E., Wainwright, S., Hailey, A., & Shannon, B. The influence of childbirth on psychiatric morbidity. *Psychological Medicine*, 1976, *6*, 297–302.
Late-date eclampsia. *Emergency Medicine*, 1980, *12*, 109–110.
Low, A. W. Postnatal treatment of toxemia. *Nursing Times*, 1975, *71*, 1671–1672.
Melchior, L. Is the postpartum period a time of crisis for some mothers? *Canadian Nurse*, 1975, *71*(7), 30–32.
Melody, G. F. Depressive reactions following hysterectomy. *American Journal of Obstetrics and Gynecology*, 1962, *83*, 410–413.
Moore, D. S., Bingham, P. R., & Keesling, O. Nursing care of the pregnant woman with diabetes mellitus. *Journal of Obstetric, Gynecologic and Neonatal Nursing*, 1981, *10*(3), 188–194.
Ms. Mid-revolutionary mores. *Ms*., 1981, *10*(1), 18.
O'Brian, B. S., & Woods, S. The paradox of DIC. *American Journal of Nursing*, 1978, *78*(11), 1878–1880.
Pitt, B. "Atypical" depression following childbirth. *British Journal of Psychiatry*, 1968, *114*, 1325–1335.
Planned Parenthood Federation of America. *Sterilization for women*. New York: Planned Parenthood Federation of America, Inc., 1978.
Rancilio, N. When a pregnant woman is diabetic: Postpartal care. *American Journal of Nursing*, 1979, *79*(3), 453–456.
Richards, D. H. Depression after hysterectomy. *Lancet*, 1973, *2*, 430–432.
Ritchie, C. A. Depression following childbirth. *Nurse Practitioner*, 1977, *2*(4), 14–17.
Schwarz, R. H., & Fruiterman, J. P. Life-threatening infections in pregnancy. *Clinical Obstetrics and Gynecology*, 1976, *19*(3), 561–575.
Stein, G., Milton, F., Bebbington, P., Wood, K., & Copper. A. Relationship between mood disturbances and free and total plasma tryptophan in postpartum women. *British Medical Journal*, 1976, *2*(6033), 457.
Tentoni, S. C., & High, K. A. Culturally induced postpartum depression. *Journal of Obstetric, Gynecologic and Neonatal Nursing*, 1980, *9*(4), 246–249.

Thomas, J. Birth of the (five week) blues. *Nursing Mirror,* 1979, *148*(34), 34.

Thompson, M. *The cry and the covenant.* New York: Signet, 1949.

Wheeler, L., & Jones, M. B. Pregnancy-induced hypertension. *Journal of Obstetric, Gynecologic and Neonatal Nursing,* 1981, *10*(3), 212–232.

Woollaston, M. Psychiatric consequences of the puerperium—some case histories. *Midwife and Health Visitor,* 1973, *9*(5), 145, 147, 149–150.

5

Parent and Infant Behaviors

Introduction

Postpartum nurses have the opportunity and responsibility for helping newly expanded families to remain in a state of precrisis. Knowledge and understanding of the developmental tasks that must be accomplished during this time enable the nurse to plan more effective care. Likewise, an awareness of attachment behaviors is necessary, so that the nurse can encourage attachment and also recognize danger signs. The Division on Maternal and Child-Health Nursing Practice of the American Nurses Association has issued a statement on parent–infant attachment (1979) that states in part: "Nurses must initiate a plan for consistent assessment of antecedent incidents and monitoring of parental attachment behavior, just as they do for assessment of physical well-being." Introducing parents to their newborn's unique features, responses, behaviors, and capabilities will help facilitate positive parent–infant interactions. As with all other aspects of maternity nursing, cultural differences must be taken into consideration when planning and delivering care.

Attachment

Attachment has been defined as a unique emotional relationship between two people which endures over time and distance (Bowlby, 1969). Bowlby first used the term *attachment* to refer to the nature of a child's tie to his or her mother. He proposed that an infant's attachment to his or her mother originates in a number of species characteristic behavior systems, becomes focused on the mother as the chief attachment figure, and serves to bind the child to the mother and the mother to the child. Bowlby identified five behavioral systems that contribute to attachment: crying and smiling, which have a signaling function and activate maternal behavior which brings the mother to the child; and sucking, following, and clinging, in which the infant takes an active role in seeking and maintaining contact. Over a period of time, Bowlby says, these systems become integrated and focused on the mother and form the basis of attachment.

Klaus and Kennell, and other of their associates, have focused on the attachment of a mother to her infant. They became interested in maternal-infant attachment in the 1960s, when they noted that after heroic measures had been used to save premature infants, these same infants would sometimes be returned to emergency rooms battered or neglected by their parents, after having been sent home thriving and intact.

Klaus and Kennell (1976) list seven principles they feel are important components in the process of attachment:

1. There is a sensitive period in the first hours of life during which it is necessary that the parents have close contact with their infant.
2. There appear to be species-specific responses to the infant in humans that appear on first contact with the infant. Characteristically, they first touch the extremities with their fingertips, trunk with fingertips, palms stroking infant, and finally encircling the infant.
3. The process of attachment is structured so that the parents will become optimally attached to only one infant at a time.
4. During the process of the mother's attachment to her infant, it is necessary that the infant respond to the mother by some signal, such as body or eye movements.
5. People who witness the birth may become attached to the infant.
6. It may be difficult to develop an attachment to one person while mourning the loss of the same or another person.
7. Early events can have long lasting effects (Klaus & Kennell, 1976, p. 14).

Many studies have been done to determine the importance of the first postpartum days and to determine what, if any, long-term effect there is from prolonged maternal–infant contact (Kennell et al., 1974; Kennell, Trause, & Klaus, 1975; Klaus et al., 1972; Klaus & Kennell, 1976; Kontos, 1978; Whiten, 1977). In general, these studies have had a control and an experimental group of women. The control group received normal hospital contact with their neonates; the experimental group had their infants in close contact early and for extended periods of time after delivery. There were significant differences between the groups at up to two years of age, with mothers in the early contact group showing more soothing, eye-to-eye contact, and fondling, suggesting that extra contact hours at birth may affect maternal behavior for at least two years.

Implicit in the work of the above researchers is that mothers who have been given extended contact with their infants show more sensitivity and are more responsive to their babies' needs. Ainsworth and others who have been studying infant–mother attachment have pointed out the importance of maternal sensitivity and responsiveness in the infant's formation of a secure attachment to its mother (Ainsworth, 1973; Ainsworth et al., 1971; Bell & Ainsworth, 1972; Blehar, Lieberman, & Ainsworth, 1977).

It should be emphasized that a great deal of research needs to be done on attachment. Numerous examples can be cited of strong attachment between adoptive parents and their infants, parents and infants who have been critically ill and separated for prolonged periods of time, women who have been seriously ill following the birth of their infants, and cases where parents and infants are separated after birth for reasons other than health. Whereas early contact seems to be important, it is obviously not the sole factor in determining the relationship that will develop between parents and infant nor is it the one determining factor in how the infant will relate to others in later life.

Lamb states that evidence thus far suggests that extended contact between women and their infants has "no clear effects on maternal behavior" (1982b, p. 767). He points out problems with many of the studies to date both in methodology and in sample differences. In another article, Lamb states that from the more than 20 projects to date, the evidence suggests that at best, maternal–infant contact has no enduring effects on either the women or their infants, although some short-term effects may be noted with some women under certain circumstances (1982a). Thus, there are many questions yet to be answered concerning the attachment process.

Little research has been done in the area of father–infant attachment, related to early contact in the postpartum period. Jones (1981) found that fathers who held their infants in the first hour of life did not differ significantly in their perceptions of their infants from fathers who did not have this early contact. She did find that the fathers with early contact showed more nonverbal behavior with their infants at one month than did those fathers without the early contact. Taubenheim (1981) found that fathers who fed their infants on the first postpartum day showed more attachment behaviors than did fathers who had not fed their infants. She concluded that engaging in caretaking activities may be important in paternal–infant bonding.

May (1982, p. 342) describes three phases of the father's involvement in pregnancy. She speculates that men who begin emotional preparation for fatherhood early, through focusing on their experience of pregnancy and redefining themselves as future fathers, may adjust more easily than those men who delay such preparation. Perry (1983, p. 208) found in her investigation no relationship between the infant's behavior and parents' perceptions of the infant. Roberts (1983, pp. 216–217) found a correlation between obligatory infant behavior (that requiring action on the part of the parents) and transition to parenthood. Her study demonstrated a difference between fathers and mothers. Fathers reported greater amounts of obligatory behavior in their infants and lower perceptions of their own role competence (parent role) than mothers. On the other hand, fathers had higher ease of transition (to parenting role) scores. Greenberg and Morris (1974) describe behavior termed engrossment (preoccupation, absorption, and interest in the infant) that characterizes the father's reaction as well as the mother's. In an extensive review of the literature on the transition to fatherhood, Hangsleben (1980) found many articles discussing the father's role, behaviors during and after pregnancy, and the impact of stress factors on fathering. In a touching essay on his experiences of fathering, McKenzie describes his feelings as he took on the role of father (1980).

More work on fathering as well as mothering needs to be done. As more and more women of infants and young children return to the work force, the father may play a more significant role in childbearing. Hangsleben (1983, p. 269) found in her investigation that fathers were very involved in infant care. Those who reported more lifestyle changes, and involvement in the care of their infants reported more signs of depression such as irritability, sleep disturbance, and fatigability, demonstrating that men as well as women experience stress and disruption when assuming the role of parent.

Implications for Nursing

What variables affect a woman's ability to assume the mothering role, and what can nurses do to facilitate this transition?

The ability to attach oneself to a child begins to develop at a very early age. The kind of mothering a woman has experienced affects what kind of mother she will become. This foundation is developed further as she progresses through her developmental course, particularly through developing interpersonal skills. A woman's self-concept can be a great help or hindrance to her maternal bonding ability. In regard to the mothering role, Rubin (1967) has identified three categories of the self-system—the ideal image, body image, and self-image—which affect a woman's attitudes and behaviors.

Having an awareness of the developmental tasks each woman needs to accomplish during this period of disequilibrium helps the nurse to plan and provide more effective care. An adolescent mother will have different concerns than will the older mother. The adolescent is suddenly confronted with the tasks of early adulthood (Havighurst, 1953), before she has had a chance to accomplish the developmental tasks of adolescence. She is probably concerned about what her peers think; she may not have become comfortable with her developing body prior to pregnancy, and now she faces the flabby postpartum figure. Other adolescents are making plans for school, jobs, moving from parents' homes. The pregnant adolescent may be forced to live with her family for several more years, or postpone her career or school plans. All of these concerns and more must be addressed if the adolescent is to assume the maternal role effectively.

The older primipara (over 30) may have a well-established career. She may be concerned about how she will manage both career and motherhood. This woman may benefit from an exploration of the possible support systems—friends, family, day care—available to her. Pointing out that even full-time mothers don't spend all of their time doing things with their children may alleviate some doubts and guilt she may have about returning to her job (Ash, 1980). The older primipara may have many outside activities she enjoys with her husband/partner. She may benefit from her nurse encouraging her to set aside "quality" time each week to spend with her mate (Malley-Corrinet, 1980). Encouraging open communication and shared parenting may help the woman discover resources she did not realize she had. By increasing her coping mechanisms in this way, the nurse enables the woman to more easily take on the maternal role.

The labor experience may affect maternal attachment. A woman in the early postpartum period must be given the opportunity to relive, verbally, her labor and delivery experience. Her body's performance is important. The birth itself begins a critical phase for the mother in relating to her infant, for she must then compare her real life infant to that of her "dream infant." If reality varies greatly with expectations, the woman will grieve the loss of her fantasized child (Clark & Affonso, 1976).

Klaus and Kennell (1976) explicitly state in their principles of attachment that "the process of attachment is structured so that parents will become optimally attached to only one infant at a time" (p. 14). This needs to be taken into consideration when a woman gives birth to more than one infant at a time. She will first attach to the "twins," attaching to each individually months later. To facilitate this attachment, the nurse should bring both twins to the mother, together, to help reinforce the fact that she has two infants (Gromada, 1981). Parents may dress twins identically to help them attach to the unit, the "twins." The nurse should observe whether the woman holds each twin close during feeding periods, and observe for other signs of disparity in attachment between the twins. Attention can tactfully be drawn to the disparity, so that the new mother can respond more appropriately (Gromada, 1981).

The Brazelton Neonatal Assessment Scale. Postpartum nurses can help new mothers (parents) become acquainted with their neonates. Blehar and associates (1977) felt that the interaction between flexible maternal response and individual infant characteristics is what leads to a secure attachment between infant and mother. The Brazelton Neonatal Behavioral Assessment Scale (1973) is a tool which is useful in demonstrating to parents the unique characteristics and capabilities of their infant. To actually perform the BNBAS, one must become certified; however, with an awareness of the content, a nurse can demonstrate to parents their child's capacity to habituate, to perform defensive maneuvers, and to organize several responses to maintain self-control. For instance, to demonstrate to parents the consolability of their infant, when the infant is crying, wait 15 seconds before intervening, to allow the infant to quiet himself. If that does not happen, use graduated measures to help the infant become quiet. First, present the face; then add the voice; then place hand on the infant's abdomen; restraining one, then both arms; holding the infant; holding and rocking; then holding, rocking, and talking to the infant. The intervention is stopped at whatever stage the infant becomes quiet.

It is important for parents to realize that infants vary in cuddliness and that they vary in degree of irritability or contentment. If parents are made aware of these individual differences, they should be better prepared to more appropriately interact with their newborns. They will be equipped to take cues from their own infant and gear their responses accordingly.

Parents need to be made aware that, at birth, their infant can turn his or her head to the human voice, prefers the human voice to other tones, can follow with his or her eyes 90 degrees a picture of the human face, but will not follow a scrambled face, and prefers milk smells over water or sugar water (Brazelton, 1979, p. 39).

The sleep or awake state of the infant must be taken into consideration when demonstrating the infant's behavioral responses. Parents benefit from this information, which enables them to plan more appropriately the timing of their interventions with their infant. The sleep and awake states used by Brazelton (1973), who used the definitions of Prechtl and Beintema (1965), consist of two sleep states and four awake states. The criteria for each state are as follows:

Sleep States

1. Deep sleep—regular breathing, eyes closed, no spontaneous activity except startles or jerky movements at regular intervals; external stimuli produce startles with some delay; suppression of startles is rapid, and state changes are less likely than from other states; no eye movements.
2. Light sleep—eyes closed; rapid eye movements can be observed under closed lids; low activity level, with random movements and startles or startle equivalents; movements are likely to be smoother and more monitored than in State One; responds to internal and external stimuli with startle equivalents, often with a resulting change of state; respirations are irregular, sucking movements occur off and on.

Awake States

3. Drowsy or semidozing—eyes may be open or closed, eyelids fluttering; activity level variable, with interspersed, mild startles from time to time; reactive to sensory stimuli, but response often delayed; state change after stimulation frequently noted; movements are usually smooth.

4. Alert—with bright look; seems to focus attention on source of stimulation, such as an object to be sucked or a visual or auditory stimulus; impinging stimuli may break through, but with some delay in response; motor activity is at a minimum.
5. Eyes open—considerable motor activity, with thrusting movements of the extremities, and even a few spontaneous startles; reactive to external stimulation with increase in startles or motor activity, but discrete reactions difficult to distinguish because of general high activity level.
6. Crying—characterized by intense crying which is difficult to break through with stimulation (from Brazelton, 1973, pp. 5–8).

The Brazelton Neonatal Behavioral Assessment Scale is made up of 27 behavioral items, which are assessed on a 9-point scale, and 20 reflex responses (Table 5.1).

The work of Barnard and colleagues contributes in an important way to screening in the neonatal period and during the first year of life (Barnard & Douglas, 1974; Barnard & Eyres, 1979).

Attachment as a Process

Attachment can be thought of as an ongoing process, rather than as a state. Few women or men feel a great love or attachment to their newborn at the instant of birth. In their earliest encounters with their infants, many mothers assume the *en face* position, first described by Robson (1967) as that position where the mother's face is rotated so that her eyes and those of the infant meet on the same vertical plane of rotation (see Figure 5.1). Eye contact appears to be very important.

Characteristically, a mother touches her infant with her finger tips, progresses to stroking with the palm, and finally encircles the infant with her arms as in Figure 5.2. Klaus, Trause, and Kennell (1975) have described this progression as happening during the first few minutes after birth, where the mother and infant are lying skin to skin. Rubin (1963) noted the same progression, but the time span was several days, rather than several minutes. The difference may have been due to the fact that the women Rubin observed were handed their infants wrapped in blankets, instead of nude.

Women progress from passively accepting their babies when

brought to them to more actively reaching and extending their fingers to receive their infants. The infant may at first be referred to as "it," then as "he/she," and finally by name. It has been found that fathers tend to refer to their infants as "it" for a longer period of time than mothers (Cogan & Edmunds, 1980). This is felt to be due to the fact that the woman has had a longer and more continuous contact with her infant than has the man, and thus it takes him longer after birth to recognize or attach to his infant.

There is a progressive interest in caretaking activities. At first the woman is satisfied to have someone else take care of both her needs and those of her infant. Rubin (1961) described the first two to three days postpartum as that of "taking-in." A postpartum hospital stay typically does not go beyond this "taking-in" stage. It is important, therefore, to include a support person—grandmother, father of baby, friend—when teaching infant care. The woman will be "taking-hold" after she leaves the hospital, taking the responsibility for infant and self-care. (Refer to Chapter 6 for teaching information.)

Women characteristically talk to their infants in a high-pitched voice and switch back to their regular voice when speaking to other adults. Infants are more receptive to high-pitched voices than lower-pitched ones (Klaus & Kennell, 1976).

Several tools are available which the postpartum nurse might find helpful in monitoring attachment. The Maternal Attachment Tool (Cropley, Lester, & Pennington, 1976) is useful in monitoring the progression of maternal–infant attachment. Using this tool may also enable the nurse to identify women who are showing a disturbance in the attachment process (Table 5.2).

A tool that can be used as a screening measure to predict the adaptive potential of a mother–infant pair is the Neonatal Perception Inventory (NPI) (Broussard, 1978) (Table 5.3). This tool is designed to be administered to women on their first or second day postpartum (Inventory I), and again when the infant is one month of age (Inventory II). This tool has the woman rate her perceptions of the "average baby" and "your baby" in areas of crying, feeding, spitting up or vomiting, sleeping, bowel movements, and patterns of eating and sleeping. Broussard (1978) notes that in our society, it is important to be better than average. This implies that when a woman rates her infant as better than average, she has a positive perception of her infant. If a woman does not rate her baby as better than average, that infant is at high risk for subsequent psychological difficulty. The next step "is to conduct a careful clinical assessment that will provide an in-depth appraisal of

Table 5.1 Behavioral and Neurological Assessment Scale

Date__________ Hour__________

Infant's name__________________ Sex___ Age________ Born_____

Mother's name______________ Father's Age____ Father's S.E.S._____

Apparent Race_______

Examiner(s)__________________ Place of Examination__________

Conditions of examination: Date of Examination__________

Birth weight_____ Current weight_____ Length_____ Head circ.___

Time examined_____ Time last fed________ Type of feeding_______

Type of delivery______________________ Apgar__________

Length of labor______________________ Birth order_________

Type, amount and timing of medication given Mother__________

____

Anesthesia?____

Abnormalities of labor_______________________________

Initial State: observe 2 minutes

1	2	3	4	5	6
deep	light	drowsy	alert	active	crying

Predominant states (mark two):

1	2	3	4	5	6

the adaptive potential of the mother–infant pair'' (Broussard, 1978, p. 57). At this point, the physician can ''establish the level of need for intervention . . . '' (Broussard, 1978, p. 57).

After the NPI is administered when the infant is one month old, the Degree of Bother Inventory (Broussard, 1978) is given to assess problems of infant behavior (Table 5.4). This covers the same topics as the NPI plus has spaces for the woman to list any other topics of concern. Since parental annoyance varies widely according to each par-

Table 5.1 (Continued)

Elicited Responses	0*	L	M	H	A
Plantar grasp		1	2	3	
Hand grasp		1	2	3	
Ankle clonus		1	2	3	
Babinski		1	2	3	
Standing		1	2	3	
Automatic walking		1	2	3	
Placing		1	2	3	
Incurvation		1	2	3	
Crawling		1	2	3	
Glabella		1	2	3	
Tonic deviation of head and eyes		1	2	3	
Nystagmus		1	2	3	
Tonic neck reflex		1	2	3	
Moro		1	2	3	
Rooting (intensity)		1	2	3	
Sucking (intensity)		1	2	3	
Passive movement					
Arms R		1	2	3	
L		1	2	3	
Legs R		1	2	3	
L		1	2	3	

Descriptive Paragraph (optional)				
Attractive	0	1	2	3
Interfering variables	0	1	2	3
Need for stimulation	0	1	2	3
What activity does he use to quiet self?				
hand to mouth				
sucking with nothing in mouth				
locking onto visual or auditory stimuli				
postural changes				
state change for no observable reason				
Comments:				

(continued)

*0 = response not elicited (omitted)

A = asymmetry

Table 5.1 (Continued)

Scale (Note State)	Initial State ____ Predominant State ____ 1 2 3 4 5 6 7 8 9
1. Response decrement to light (2, 3)	
2. Response decrement to rattle (2, 3)	
3. Response decrement to bell (2, 3)	
4. Response decrement to pinprick (1, 2, 3)	
5. Orientation inanimate visual (4 only)	
6. Orientation inanimate auditory (4, 5)	
7. Orientation animate visual (4 only)	
8. Orientation animate auditory (4, 5)	
9. Orientation animate visual and auditory (4 only)	
10. Alertness (4 only)	
11. General tonus (4, 5)	
12. Motor maturity (4, 5)	
13. Pull-to-sit (3, 5)	
14. Cuddliness (4, 5)	
15. Defensive movements (4)	
16. Consolability (6 to 5, 4, 3, 2)	
17. Peak of excitement (6)	
18. Rapidity of buildup (from 1, 2 to 6)	

Table 5.1 (Continued)

Scale (Note State)	Initial State ______ Predominant State ______ 1 2 3 4 5 6 7 8 9
19. Irritability (3, 4, 5)	______
20. Activity (alert states)	______
21. Tremulousness (all states)	______
22. Startle (3, 4, 5, 6)	______
23. Lability of skin color (from 1 to 6)	______
24. Lability of states (all states)	______
25. Self-quieting activity (6, 5 to 4, 3, 2, 1)	______
26. Hand-mouth facility (all states)	______

Used with permission. From Brazelton, T. B. (1973), Neonatal Behavioral Assessment Scale, Clinics in Developmental Medicine No. 50. London: SIMP with Heinemann Medical; Philadelphia: Lippincott.

ent's emotional orientation toward the child, the decision as to what constitutes a problem varies among parents. The Degree of Bother Inventory is scored by totaling the values of each answer (1 through 4). A score of 24 would indicate that the woman is easily annoyed by her child, a score of 6 that she's not bothered at all.

In a longitudinal study, the NPI at one month was predictive of emotional disorder in children at age four and a half. The NPI at one to two days postpartum was not predictive of the child's emotional development at age four and a half (Broussard & Hartner, 1970). At age 10 to 11 there was again a statistically significant relationship between the one-month NPI and the emotional development of the children (Broussard, 1979).

The Denver Developmental Screening Test (DDST) (Frankenberg & Dodds, 1967) can be used by a trained examiner as a screening tool for detection of developmental delay in infants and children. This screen-

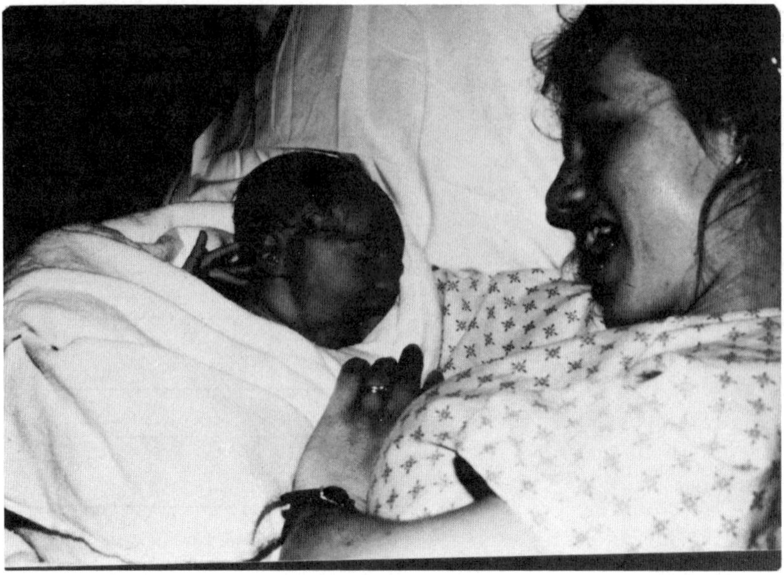

Figure 5.1 *En face* position. (Photograph by Douglas C. Beck.)

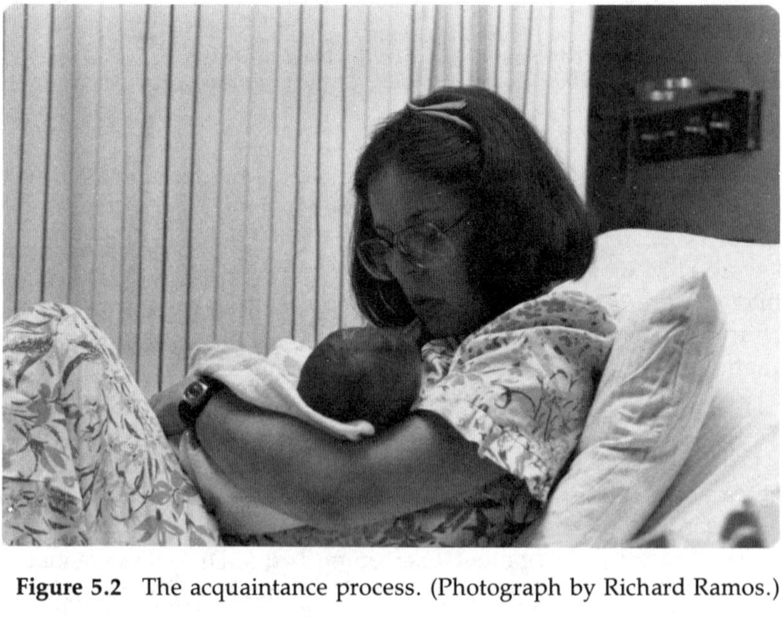

Figure 5.2 The acquaintance process. (Photograph by Richard Ramos.)

ing test covers personal-social, fine motor-adaptive, language, and gross motor areas of development. The DDST can be used with parents to give them anticipatory guidance as to what they might expect of their infant, developmentally, over a time period, in addition to encouraging parents to provide appropriate stimulation for their infants.

Parenting

Assumption of the parenting role is one of the developmental hazardous events affecting individuals and families during the puerperium. Encouraging attachment behaviors, demonstrating the infant's unique behaviors and capabilities to the parents, and assessing parents' perceptions of their infants are done in anticipation that this focus of care will be the beginning of successful parenting. Parenting in our contemporary American society can be difficult. In general, the extended family of the past is just that. The mother–father–child/children may live many miles away from their nearest relative. The burden of parenting is no longer shared by other adult relatives (Clark, 1981).

Assessment

The postpartum assessment should include an assessment of parenting capabilities. This should include caretaking skills (see Chapter 6) as well as the emotional or affective component of parenting. Each woman should be observed for the attachment behaviors discussed earlier (e.g., reaching, touching, *en face* positioning, eye-to-eye contact, and pronominalization) as well as for rhythm-reciprocity patterns. Brazelton (1974) described an infant cycle of interaction to which sensitive mothers respond.

Curry found in her study (1983, p. 119) that women vary in their ability to adapt to motherhood. In addition to previous experience with infants, help from husbands and postpartum nurses and self-concept were important to adaptation.

Wilson (1978) points out that parenting classes often teach child development and child care skills, without first ascertaining whether parents have a "foundation" for parenting. She emphasizes the importance of assessing the parenting the parents received, the level of the parents' interpersonal skills, and the support systems available to them.

In assessing the woman's support systems, the husband/father of the baby should be given priority consideration. Does the woman feel he will be helpful, does she feel close to him, does he express concern

Table 5.2 Maternal Attachment Tool

Name________________ Delivery Date___________ Today's Date_________

	Circle points for observed behavior
I. Identifying behaviors: The mother's observing or inquiring about her infant to gain knowledge of infant's appearance, wholeness, and state of function	
A. Appearance and function	
1. Makes reference to sex of the infant, e.g., "He's going to be a football player," or gets infant a sex-linked toy.	+1
2. Makes reference to size of the infant, e.g., "She's so little."	+1
3. Inspects or reviews baby's body features (hair, fingers, face, feet, and other parts of body).	+1
4. Asks questions or makes statements pertaining to wholeness of the infant, e.g., "Is he all right?" or "Well, he has all ten toes."	+1
5. Verbally questions or comments on body functions of baby, e.g., "Look, she's wet," or "Look at him move!"	+1
I-A score (total circled points):	
B. Appraisal of infant's condition	
6. Asks no questions about baby's condition	0
7. Makes unrealistic statements (optimistic or pessimistic) regarding baby's condition, e.g., saying skin looks better when it looks worse.	-1
8. Asks brief questions about baby's condition, e.g., "How's he eating?" or "How much weight has he gained?"	+1
9. Asks realistic questions or makes realistic comments about infant's condition with specific references to such things as skin, scalp, eyes, face, circumcision, and cord in the normal newborn or IV, monitor, bilirubin lights, and physical symptoms (e.g., jaundice or color) in the high-risk infant.	+2

Table 5.2 (Continued)

	Circle points for observed behavior
10. Verbal statements by mother that denote her awareness of changes in the baby's condition, e.g., "She is breathing more slowly today," or "His skin doesn't look as dry today."	+3
I-B score (total circled points):	
II. Locating behaviors: Cognitively determining the baby's position within the sphere of her significant social system	
A. Verbally associates infant with an animal or animal characteristics.	0
B. Associates infant with inanimate object.	0
C. Associates infant's characteristics with human characteristics, e.g., "He looks like an old man," or "She looks more like a real baby now."	+1
D. Associates infant's characteristics with other family members, e.g., "She has her daddy's big feet," or "She looks just like her sister."	+2
II score (Do not total: record highest circled score):	____
III. Modalities of interaction: The method through which the mother begins to relate to her baby, using visual, verbal, and tactile behaviors	
A. Verbal contact	
1. Mother talks or sings to baby.	+1
2. Mother uses infant's given name when talking to baby.	+1
B. Visual contact	
3. Establishes position en face.	+1
4. Talks about baby's opening eyes; verbally encourages this.	+1
5. Stimulates infant to open eyes by shading them from the light, changing position, and other maneuvers.	+1

(continued)

Table 5.2 (Continued)

	Circle points for observed behavior
C. Tactile-kinaesthetic contact	
6. Touches extremities or head.	+1
7. Extends touch to trunk of baby's body.	+2
8. Fingertip touch.	+1
9. Finger touch (stroking).	+1
10. Palm contact.	+2
11. Draws infant to trunk of her body (body contact).	+1
12. Snuggles baby to shoulder with cheek-to-cheek contact.	+2
13. Spontaneous movements initiated by mother to increase her contact with baby, e.g., patting, kissing, cuddling, rocking, playing, and soothing.	+1
III score (total circled points):	____
IV. <u>Caretaking behaviors</u>: Activities of mother aimed at supporting and protecting infant to foster child's optimal growth and development	
A. Participation in care	
1. No participation in baby's care.	0
2. Holds infant but performs no care tasks.	+1
3. Recognizes infant's needs but leaves solution up to nurse, e.g., "Oh, the baby's wet."	+2
4. Communicates baby's need to nurse and asks if she can do the task, e.g., "She's wet; can I change her?"	+3
5. Performs isolated aspects of care such as changing diapers and feeding baby but needs encouragement from staff.	+4
6. Recognizes baby's needs and performs appropriate interventions, e.g., bathing, changing, and giving medication.	+5

Table 5.2 (Continued)

	Circle points for observed behavior
IV-A score (Do not total: record highest circled score):	____
B. Planning home care	
7. Makes no reference to baby's discharge or to care that infant will require at home.	0
8. Refers to baby's eventual discharge or to care that infant will require at home.	+1
9. Asks questions in preparation for infant's discharge, e.g., "What kind of soap should I use?" or "When is the best time to give the bath at home?"	+2
10. Makes reference to preparing for discharge actively, e.g., "We've just finished her room," or "I bought everything but the bottles today."	+3
IV-B score (Do not total: record highest circled score):	____
Scores for each section: I-A ____	
I-B ____	
II ____	
III ____	
IV-A ____	
IV-B ____	
Total maternal attachment score	____
Length of visits by mother to hospitalized infant	____
1. None	
2. 1 to 15 minutes	
3. 16 to 30 minutes	
4. 31 to 60 minutes	

(continued)

Table 5.2 (Continued)

	Circle points for observed behavior
5. 61 to 120 minutes	
6. Over 2 hours	
<u>Frequency of visits by mother to hospitalized infant</u>	____
1. None	
2. Once a day	
3. Twice a day	
4. Three times a day	
5. More than three times a day	
<u>Frequency of calls to hospital by mother</u>	____
1. None	
2. Once a day	
3. Twice a day	
4. Three times a day	
5. More than three times a day	

Used with permission. Reproduced from Cropley, Catherine, Lester, Priscilla, & Pennington, Sharon, Assessment tool for measuring maternal attachment behaviors. In McNall, Leota Lester, and Galeener, Janet Trask (Editors), <u>Current Practice in Obstetric and Gynecologic Nursing</u>, Vol. I. St. Louis, 1976, The C. V. Mosby Co.

about her, interest in his infant? In talking with the father of the baby, ask whether he has had experience with children, whether he enjoyed taking care of and being around small children, whether he desires more children. What does he know about baby care? All of these factors have been found to influence fathers' attitudes (Leonard, 1976). If the father of the baby is no longer in the picture, ascertain to whom the woman goes with problems, to whom does she feel close, on whom can she count for help (Josten, 1981).

Also to be assessed is the mother's physical and emotional energy (Bishop, 1976). A woman who has an infection, chronic disease, or even a low hemoglobin level may not have the energy to adapt to and parent a newborn. Emotional energy is somewhat more difficult to assess during a short postpartum stay but does need to be considered. Listen to what she says—are her comments about herself and/or her infant more negative than positive (Bishop, 1976)? Only after the parents' strengths and weaknesses are assessed can the health professional assist in areas of need.

Nurse's Role in Augmentation of Parenting

If the nurse is working in an institution whose maternity service practices family-centered nursing, fathers, along with the mothers, should be included in infant-care classes and discussion groups. If the father of the infant is no longer a significant person, the woman's support person (mother, sister, friend) should be included in any instructional or discussion groups. If the institution does not practice family-centered care, the nurse should work toward implementing that change (refer to Chapter 8).

Family-centered nursing implies the involvement of siblings, if present. Many institutions now allow some degree of sibling involvement. Parents who have at least one other child at home are usually concerned about jealousy and welcome the opportunity to discuss this concern. They may benefit from knowing that jealousy is to be expected. Siblings should be encouraged to interact with and participate in the care of the infant, as this involvement may promote the development of attachment, just as it does with an adult (Vestal, 1979). Wranesh (1982) found that postnatal infection rates were not significantly increased by visits from well siblings. Sibling visitation to the hospital is an important aspect of family-centered care (Kraus, 1979). Big sister in Figure 5.3 is getting acquainted with her new baby brother.

Having regularly scheduled parent (mother/father or mother/significant other) discussion groups in which infant characteristics, behaviors, and rhythms are discussed may help the new parents to have more realistic perceptions of their infants, and therefore be better prepared to interact positively with them. The importance of promptly responding to their infants' cries should be emphasized, as that has been found to influence the development in the infant of noncrying forms of communication.

Table 5.3 Neonatal Perception Inventory I. Average Baby

How much crying do you think the average baby does?

a great deal	a good bit	moderate amount	very little	none

How much trouble do you think the average baby has in feeding?

a great deal	a good bit	moderate amount	very little	none

How much spitting up or vomiting do you think the average baby does?

a great deal	a good bit	moderate amount	very little	none

How much difficulty do you think the average baby has in sleeping?

a great deal	a good bit	moderate amount	very little	none

How much difficulty does the average baby have with bowel movements?

a great deal	a good bit	moderate amount	very little	none

How much trouble do you think the average baby has in settling down to a predictable pattern of eating and sleeping?

a great deal	a good bit	moderate amount	very little	none

Broussard, E. R., Psychosocial disorders in children: Early assessment of infants at risk, Continuing Education for the Family Physician, February 1978, Volume 8, Number 2, 44-57.

Encouraging the family unit to be together as much as possible during the postpartum period helps the man and woman become acquainted with and feel comfortable with their newborn. Rooming-in may have a positive influence on later parenting (O'Conner et al., 1978). Fathers need opportunities to become acquainted with their infants, too, as in Figure 5.4.

Postpartum nurses need to be aware of the community resources available to parents. Visiting nurse services can be an invaluable aid to new parents. Because of the abbreviated postpartum stay, most women are discharged while still in the "taking-in" phase (Rubin, 1961)

Table 5.3 (Continued) Neonatal Perception Inventory I. Your Baby

How much crying do you think your baby will do?

a great deal	a good bit	moderate amount	very little	none

How much trouble do you think your baby will have feeding?

a great deal	a good bit	moderate amount	very little	none

How much spitting up or vomiting do you think your baby will do?

a great deal	a good bit	moderate amount	very little	none

How much difficulty do you think your baby will have sleeping?

a great deal	a good bit	moderate amount	very little	none

How much difficulty do you expect your baby to have with bowel movements?

a great deal	a good bit	moderate amount	very little	none

How much trouble do you think that your baby will have settling down to a predictable pattern of eating and sleeping?

a great deal	a good bit	moderate amount	very little	none

(continued)

and would probably benefit from a community nurse's visit during the "taking-hold" phase.

If parenting classes are available in the community, make this known to the new parents. If these classes are not available, the health professional might consider organizing such a support group. Stranik and Hogberg (1979) reported on a parent program which included a parent support group that met for four weekly sessions, beginning when the infants were between one and four weeks old. The sessions, which covered topics ranging from resolution of the labor experience through long-range needs of the infant, were well received by the parents. These group sessions were run jointly by a maternity and a pediatric nurse.

Table 5.3 (Continued) Neonatal Perception Inventory II. Average Baby

How much crying do you think the average baby does?

a great deal	a good bit	moderate amount	very little	none

How much trouble do you think the average baby has in feeding?

a great deal	a good bit	moderate amount	very little	none

How much spitting up or vomiting do you think the average baby does?

a great deal	a good bit	moderate amount	very little	none

How much difficulty do you think the average baby has in sleeping?

a great deal	a good bit	moderate amount	very little	none

How much difficulty does the average baby have with bowel movements?

a great deal	a good bit	moderate amount	very little	none

How much trouble do you think the average baby has in settling down to a predictable pattern of eating and sleeping?

a great deal	a good bit	moderate amount	very little	none

Cultural Aspects

In order for nurses to provide postpartum care which will promote attachment and successful parenting among our client population, consideration should be given to the cultural background from which the client comes. Most institutions serve populations which are made up of only a few ethnic or cultural groups. It is realistic, therefore, for us to become knowledgeable about the beliefs and customs of the population which we serve. It is important, too, to determine whether a particular client subscribes to the beliefs of her ethnic group, or whether her values have become "Americanized."

Table 5.3 (Continued) Neonatal Perception Inventory II. Your Baby

How much crying has your baby done?

a great deal	a good bit	moderate amount	very little	none

How much trouble has your baby had feeding?

a great deal	a good bit	moderate amount	very little	none

How much spitting up or vomiting has your baby done?

a great deal	a good bit	moderate amount	very little	none

How much difficulty has your baby had in sleeping?

a great deal	a good bit	moderate amount	very little	none

How much difficulty has your baby had with bowel movements?

a great deal	a good bit	moderate amount	very little	none

How much trouble has your baby had in settling down to a predictable pattern of eating and sleeping?

a great deal	a good bit	moderate amount	very little	none

The Afro-American woman has experienced many difficulties and knows her child will face many hardships. Little value, therefore, is placed on behaviors that are felt to "spoil" the child. Picking up and soothing the baby is done judiciously, for the baby must learn early to cope (Carrington, 1978). Love is expressed during physical caretaking activities and at feeding times. A "good" black mother may be equated with one who successfully feeds her baby; these women may become frustrated when their infants fall asleep at a feeding time before they have taken much formula or nursed for very long. The nurse may gently explain to the black woman the need for cuddling, for being responsive to her infant's cry. Explaining newborn eating patterns may help

Table 5.4 Degree of Bother Inventory

Crying	a great deal	somewhat	very little	none
Spitting up or vomiting	a great deal	somewhat	very little	none
Sleeping	a great deal	somewhat	very little	none
Feeding	a great deal	somewhat	very little	none
Elimination	a great deal	somewhat	very little	none
Lack of a predictable schedule	a great deal	somewhat	very little	none
Other (specify):				
________________	a great deal	somewhat	very little	none
________________	a great deal	somewhat	very little	none
________________	a great deal	somewhat	very little	none
________________	a great deal	somewhat	very little	none

alleviate the woman's frustration and make the postpartum days more satisfying for her (Carrington, 1978).

There are many Arab Americans in the United States, mainly from Palestine, Lebanon, Egypt, Iraq, and Yemen (Meleis & Sorrell, 1981). Many Arab values and customs differ greatly from those of contemporary Western societies, including that of the United States. Arab women generally do not have layettes prior to delivery. This should not be taken as evidence of a lack of interest in the infant. Planning ahead is seen as possibly defying God's will. Not planning ahead also avoids disappointment. Children, especially sons, are highly valued, and it is important that the family be together at occasions such as a birth (Meleis & Sorrell, 1981).

The traditional Mexican American family is a large one, and the Mexican American child receives much attention from his or her many siblings. Other adult relatives may be named co-parent and sponsor the infant for baptism. Relatives may even "adopt" and raise the child, which can be helpful to a woman feeling overwhelmed by many children (Kay, 1978).

The extended family and a love of children are values held by traditional Puerto Ricans (Sanavitis & Murillo-Rohde, 1978). Traditionally, Puerto Rican girls have married and borne children at a very early age. The maternal grandmother generally is with her daughter to do most of the child care. In large families, the older children help with

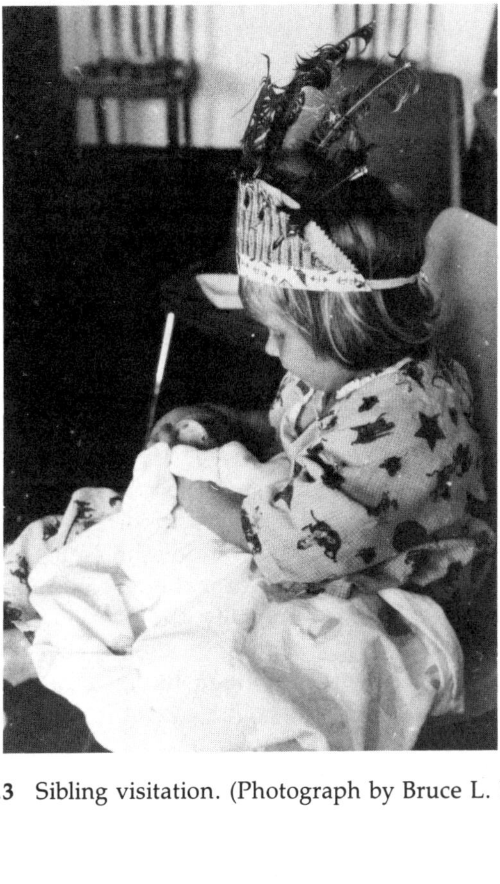

Figure 5.3 Sibling visitation. (Photograph by Bruce L. Beck.)

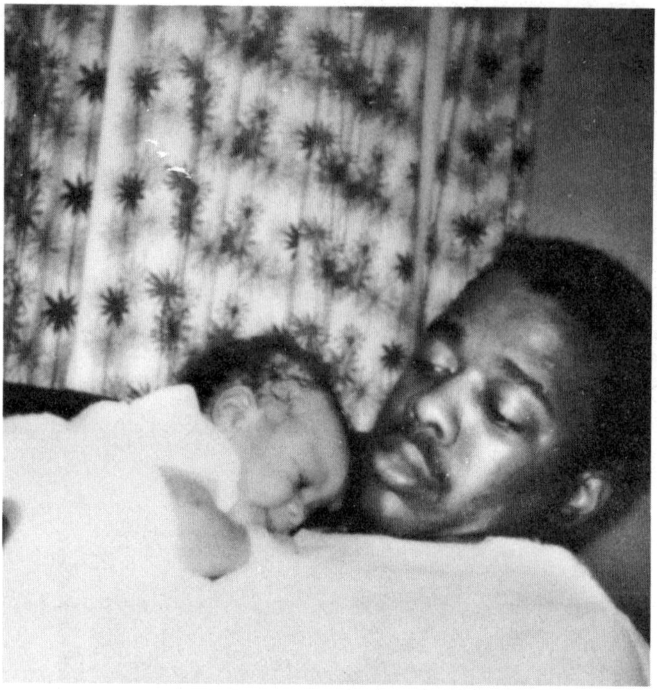

Figure 5.4 Getting acquainted. (Photograph by Marie Knight.)

the younger ones, as well as with the housework. When there is no extended family to help in the postpartum period, the husband may help at home, although this "woman's work" has not traditionally been done by men (Sanavitis & Murillo-Rohde, 1978).

The Vietnamese have been one of the more recent groups to enter the United States in large numbers. Their Southeast Asian culture is quite different from ours, and many misunderstandings have occurred as a result of this gap. Families are very important in the life of the Vietnamese, with sons being valued over daughters. If a couple is without a biological son, it is not unusual for them to adopt a son or son-in-law (Stringfellow, 1978). Traditionally, the Vietnamese mother has her infant with her constantly. The infant's slightest cry is tended to without delay. In immigrant families, the maternal grandmother plays a key role in childrearing, so that the mother can return to work (Stringfellow, 1978).

These cultural differences are examples of the diversity to be found across the United States. It is the responsibility of the nurse to become familiar with the values and beliefs of these cultural groups that she or he serves.

Summary

Infants come uniquely equipped to signal their needs to those around them. We must be prepared to demonstrate those infant abilities for new parents, so that they are better prepared to interact with and attach to their infant (Brazelton, 1979). In our contemporary society of nuclear families, new parents lack the support system provided by the extended families of the past. We need to explore, with these parents, ways in which they can maintain their equilibrium during this unsettling time.

The United States is a culturally diverse country. Nurses must make the effort to learn about the cultural beliefs and values of those with whom they work. Childrearing, or parenting, practices vary greatly among the different cultural groups (Clark, 1981).

References

Ainsworth, M. D. S. The development of infant-mother attachment. In B. Caldwell & H. Riccuiti (Eds.), *Review of child development research* (Vol. 3). Chicago: University of Chicago Press, 1973.

Ainsworth, M. D. S., Blehar, M. C., Waters, E., & Wall, S. *Patterns of attachment: A psychological study of the strange situation.* New Jersey: Lawrence Erlbaum, 1971.

Ash, M. J. Working and parenting: Can we do both? *Issues in Health Care of Women*, 1980, *2*(1), 15–23.

Barnard, K. E., & Douglas, H. B. (Eds.). *Child health assessment. Part 1: A literature review.* Bethesda, Md.: U.S. Department of Health, Education and Welfare, 1974.

Barnard, K. E., & Eyres, S. J. (Eds.). *Child health assessment. Part 2: The first year of life.* Hyattsville, Md.: U.S. Department of Health, Education and Welfare, 1979.

Bell, S. M., & Ainsworth, M. D. S. Infant crying and maternal responsiveness. *Child Development*, 1972, *43*(4), 1171–1190.

Bishop, B. A guide to assessing parenting capabilities. *American Journal of Nursing*, 1976, *76*(11), 1784–1787.

Blehar, M. D., Lieberman, A. F., & Ainsworth, M. D. S. Early face-to-face interaction and its relation to later infant attachment. *Child Development*, 1977, *48*, 182–194.

Bowlby, J. *Attachment.* New York: Basic Books, 1969.

Brazelton, T. B. *The neonatal behavioral assessment scale.* Philadelphia: Lippincott, 1973.

Brazelton, T. B. The origins of reciprocity: The early mother-infant interaction. In M. Lewis & L. A. Rosenblum (Eds.), *Origins of behavior: The effect of the infant on its caregiver.* New York: John Wiley & Sons, 1974.

Brazelton, T. B. Behavioral competence of the newborn infant. *Seminars in Perinatology,* 1979, *3*(1), 35–44.

Broussard, E. R., Psychosocial disorders in children: Early assessment of infants at risk. *Continuing Education for the Family Physician,* February 1978, *8*(2), 44–57.

Broussard, E. R. Assessment of the adaptive potential of the mother–infant system: The neonatal perception inventories. *Seminars in Perinatology,* 1979, *3*(1), 91–100.

Broussard, E. R., & Hartner, M. S. Maternal perception of the neonate as related to development. *Child Psychiatry and Human Development,* 1970, *1,* 16–25.

Carrington, B. W. The Afro-American. In A. Clark (Ed.), *Culture childbearing health professionals.* Philadelphia: Davis, 1978.

Clark, A. L. *Culture and childrearing.* Philadelphia: Davis, 1981.

Clark, A. L., & Affonso, D. D. Infant behavior and maternal attachment: Two sides of the coin. *American Journal of Maternal Child Nursing,* 1976, March-April, 94–100.

Cogan, R., & Edmunds, E. P. Pronominalization: A linguistic facet of the maternal-paternal sensitive period. *Nursing Research,* 1980, *29*(4), 225–227.

Curry, M. A. Variables related to adaptation to motherhood in "normal" primiparous women. *Journal of Obstetric, Gynecologic, and Neonatal Nursing,* 1983, *12*(2), 115–121.

Cropley, C., Lester, P., & Pennington, S. Assessment tool for measuring maternal attachment behaviors. In L. K. McNall & J. T. Galeener (Eds.), *Current practice in obstetric and gynecologic nursing* (Vol. 1). St. Louis: Mosby, 1976.

Division of Maternal and Child Health Nursing Practice. *Statement on parental-infant attachment.* Kansas City, Mo.: American Nurses Association, 1979.

Frankenburg, W. K., & Dodds, J. B. The Denver developmental screening test. *Journal of Pediatrics,* 1967, *71,* August, 181–191.

Greenberg, M., & Morris, N. Engrossment: The newborn's impact upon the father. *American Journal of Orthopsychiatry,* 1974, *44,* 520–531.

Gromada, K. Maternal-infants attachment: The first step toward individualizing twins. *American Journal of Maternal Child Nursing,* 1981, *6*(2), 129–134.

Hangsleben, K. L. Transition to fatherhood: Literature review. *Issues in Health Care of Women,* 1980, *2*(5–6), 81–97.

Hangsleben, K. L. Transition to fatherhood: An exploratory study. *Journal of Obstetric, Gynecologic, and Neonatal Nursing,* 1983, *12*(4), 265–270.

Havighurst, R. *Human development and education.* New York: McKay, 1953.

Jones, C. Father to infant attachment: Effects of early contact and characteristics of the infant. *Research in Nursing and Health,* 1981, *4,* 193–200.

Joston, L. Prenatal assessment guide for illuminating possible problems with parenting. *American Journal of Maternal Child Nursing*, 1981, *6*(2), 113–117.

Kay, M. A. The Mexican American. In A. Clark (Ed.), *Culture childbearing health professionals*. Philadelphia: Davis, 1978.

Kennell, J. H., Jerauld, R., Wolfe, H., Chesler, D., Kreger, N. C., McAlpine, W., Steffa, M., & Klaus, M. H. Maternal behavior one year after early and extended postpartum contact. *Developmental Medicine and Child Neurology*, 1974, *16*, 172–180.

Kennell, J. H., Trause, M. A., & Klaus, M. H. Evidence for a sensitive period in the human mother. In *Parent infant interaction*. Ciba Foundation Symposium No. 33, Amsterdam: Elsvier, 1975.

Klaus, M. H., Jerauld, R., Kreger, N. C., McAlpine, W., Steffa, M., & Kennell, J. H. Maternal attachment: Importance of the first postpartum days. *The New England Journal of Medicine*, 1972, *286*, 460–463.

Klaus, M. H., & Kennell, J. H. *Maternal-infant bonding: The impact of early separation or loss on family development*. St. Louis: Mosby, 1976.

Klaus, M. H., Trause, M. A., & Kennell, J. H. Does human maternal behavior after delivery show a characteristic pattern? In *Parent infant interaction*. Ciba Foundation Symposium No. 33, Amsterdam: Elsvier, 1975.

Kontos, D. A study of the effects of extended mother-infant contact on maternal behavior at one and three months. *Birth and the Family Journal*, 1978, *5*(3), 133–140.

Kraus, H. Postpartum hospital visits for children. *Issues in Health Care of Women*, 1979, *1*(4), 27–39.

Lamb, M. E. The bonding phenomenon: Misinterpretations and their implications. *Journal of Pediatrics*, 1982, *101*(4), 555–557. (a)

Lamb, M. E. Early contact and maternal-infant bonding: One decade later. *Pediatrics*, 1982, *70*(5), 763–768. (b)

Leonard, S. W. How first-time fathers feel toward their newborns. *American Journal of Maternal Child Nursing*, 1976, *1*(6), 361–365.

Malley-Corrinet, A. Marriage-motherhood-career: The triangle of constant responsibility. *Issues in Health Care of Women*, 1980, *2*(1), 37–47.

May, K. A. Three phases of father involvement in pregnancy. *Nursing Research*, 1982, *31*(6), 337–342.

McKenzie, R. A. The road to fatherhood: One man's personal remembrances. *Issues in Health Care of Women*, 1980, *2*(5–6), 99–106.

Meleis, A. I., & Sorrell, L. Arab American women and their birth experiences. *American Journal of Maternal Child Nursing*, 1981, *6*(3), 171–176.

O'Connor, S., Sherrod, K. B., Sandler, H. M., & Veitze, P. M. The effect of extended postpartum contact on problems with parenting: A controlled study of 301 families. *Birth and the Family Journal*, 1978, *5*(4), 231–234.

Perry, S. E. Parents' perceptions of their newborn following structured interactions. *Nursing Research*, 1983, *32*(4), 208–212.

Prechtl, H., & Beintema, D. L. *The neurological examination of the full-term newborn infant*. London: The Spastics International Medical Publications in association with William Heinemann Ltd., 1965.

Roberts, F. B. Infant behavior and the transition to parenthood. *Nursing Research*, 1983, *32*(4), 213–217.

Robson, K. S. The role of eye-to-eye contact in maternal-infant attachment. *Journal of Child Psychology, Psychiatry, and Allied Disciplines*, 1967, *8*, 13–25.

Rubin, R. Basic maternal behavior. *Nursing Outlook*, 1961, *9*, 683–686.

Rubin, R. Maternal touch. *Nursing Outlook*, 1963, *11*, 828–831.

Rubin, R. Attainment of the maternal role. Part I. Process. *Nursing Research*, 1967, *16*, 237–245.

Sanavitis, A. M., & Murillo-Rohde, I. The Puerto Rican. In A. Clark (Ed.), *Culture childbearing health professionals*. Philadelphia: Davis, 1978.

Stranik, M. K., & Hogberg, B. L. Transition into parenthood. *American Journal of Nursing*, 1979, January, 90–93.

Stringfellow, L. The Vietnamese. In A. Clark (Ed.), *Culture childbearing health professionals*. Philadelphia: Davis, 1978.

Taubenheim, A. M. Paternal-infant bonding in the first-time father. *Journal of Obstetric, Gynecologic, and Neonatal Nursing*, 1981, *10*(4), 261–264.

Vestal, K. W. Siblings: Adapting to accommodate the neonate. *Issues in Health Care of Women*, 1979, *1*(4), 13–25.

Whiten, A. Assessing the effects of prenatal events on the success of the mother-infant relationship. In H. R. Schaffer (Ed.), *Studies in mother-infant interaction*. New York: Academic Press, 1977.

Wilson, A. L. Parenting in perspective. *Family Community Health*, 1978, November, 65–77.

Wranesh, B. L. The effect of sibling visitation on bacterial colonization rate in neonates. *Journal of Obstetric, Gynecologic, and Neonatal Nursing*, 1982, *11*(4), 211–213.

6

Teaching and Learning Needs

Introduction

The goal of the nurse during the hospitalized portion of postpartum is to provide parents with the information they need to care for themselves and to begin to care for their infants. The time allowed for this teaching to take place is becoming shorter. Women leave the hospital with their newborns as early as eight hours postpartum. Often there is no extended family available to provide support in the home. This chapter addresses the teaching and learning needs of parents during postpartum. Anticipatory guidance will equip parents to cope with the many tasks to be accomplished during this time and, therefore, to remain in precrisis.

Assessment

Nursing augmentation and intervention must be based on assessment of needs and readiness to learn. The assessment done during the immediate postpartum period must be expanded to include the parents' knowledge about the developmental hazardous events they will be facing. Parents have varying degrees of knowledge deficits regarding biophysical and psychosocial self-care and infant care. Sumner and Fritsch (1977) found parents' concerns to be about the infant's needs and behaviors. Gruis (1977) found the woman's concerns to be centered about restoring her figure and integrating a new family member. Role assumption and role conflict were identified as problems in Sheehan's (1981) study.

Collecting the data base may be helped by assessment tools or guides (Bishop, 1980, Chap. 10; Campbell & Smith, 1977; Schmidt, 1978). Age, parity, and marital status are factors that affect the woman's perception of the birth event as well as her perception of her postpartum needs. The unwed adolescent parent may have different psychosocial needs for resources than the 34-year-old married parent (Howley, 1981). The primiparous woman may need more information than her multiparous counterpart, but she may have had experiences which will have provided her with coping mechanisms. Some primiparas have cared for much younger siblings or nieces and nephews. Perhaps the woman has extensive babysitting experience or has been the support person for a friend or relative with a new baby. Other women have had little or no contact with infants and children. Many childbirth education classes have an infant care class during the prenatal period. Parents who have attended these classes bring a certain amount of knowledge with them to postpartum. Asking the woman what preparations she has made at home for the infant will also provide data from which assessment and plans can be drawn.

Primiparas may have no knowledge of the characteristics of lochia or of the involution process. Previous use of tampons or peri pads and general perineal hygiene concepts will influence the learning needs. Contraceptive history is an important piece of data. The woman's perception of her sexual functioning and her past experiences, if any, with birth control begin to determine the extent of the teaching needs.

Multiparas have had different experiences. Assessment of their needs includes the number, ages, and sex of the other children, their previous infant feeding methods, and the perception of their previous childbearing experiences. Contraceptive history and previous sexual adjustment may have different teaching implications. Sibling rivalry and family integration are concerns for these parents (Gruis, 1977).

The learning needs for self-care and infant care are affected by the type of delivery experience. Cesarean delivery, planned or unplanned, is a situational hazardous event which has impact on the postpartum experience. Assessment of the woman's perception of the event and her biophysical and psychosocial coping mechanisms and supports are essential for planning appropriate interventions. Women who have undergone a postpartum sterilization procedure add another dimension to self-care needs.

Fathers are all too often ignored members of families. The postpartum nurse who practices from a family-centered perspective realizes that fathers can be a resource and support for the woman (Gruis, 1977). Fathers have needs of their own to meet for integrating their new roles (Cronenwett & Kunst-Wilson, 1981). More research has recently been focused on the development of the paternal–infant bond (Greenberg & Morris, 1974; Taubenheim, 1981). Men have also had varying experiences with infants. In this society the nurse must be aware that the man may biologically be a first-time father even though the woman may be a multipara or the man may have fathered other children while the woman is a primipara. Assessment of how much involvement the father wishes to have during the hospitalization and of how much he will be available at home for support affects the planning for teaching.

Identification of additional or other supports and resources which will be available at home is also part of the assessment process. The lack of available extended family has had the impact on the postpartum period of isolating women at home during the puerperium. Rubin (1975, p. 1684) characterizes the postpartal period as ''unbelievably cruel'' and ''most vulnerable.'' Ascertaining whether someone will be available for the woman during this time when professional help is not readily available is an important factor in the assessment of needs.

As discussed in Chapter 3, the cultural aspects must be taken into account during every step of assessment. The nurse must be familiar with the customs and beliefs toward the puerperium of the different cultural groups which are a part of the client population. One important aspect of assessment for cultural differences is whether that particular woman ascribes to the norms of her culture or ethnic background.

Once the data base of assessment is completed, the diagnosis of knowledge deficit can be made for each area of need. If based on the data collected, the assessment will be individual and unique for that parent's needs, although many needs will be similar to those of other postpartum clients.

Planning Interventions

When the nursing diagnosis for specific knowledge deficits is made, planning interventions with the woman and her family can begin. Most knowledge deficits can be identified as biophysical for self-care and infant care, and psychosocial for self-care and infant care. Although the biophysical and psychosocial aspects of self-care and infant care overlap, each will be treated as a separate entity for purposes of discussion.

Teaching Strategies

Planning interventions include choosing from a variety of teaching methods which are age and need appropriate. There should be options for individual or group classes. Croog and Zigrossi (1983) describe parenting luncheons on a postpartum unit as a vehicle for instructing women and their spouses (if present) on various aspects of parenthood and infant care. This is one innovative approach to teaching parents in a relaxed, social atmosphere. Judicious use of instructional media can benefit both nurse and client. Slide–tape presentations can often be viewed in the woman's room at her convenience. Closed-circuit television or videotapes can be scheduled for viewing at times when the unit activity is low. Some topics that lend themselves to instructional media include baby bath demonstrations, formula preparation, breast self-exam, and family planning methods. Care must be taken that these tools do not replace the nurse as a resource to answer questions and provide guidance and individual teaching when necessary.

The majority of postpartum parents are adult learners. As such they can be self-directed and goal oriented (Knowles, 1970). Schmidt (1978) describes a teaching guide which lets parents decide what they need to know. Providing options on how to get the information gives them or reinforces their feeling of control. Because the woman is "taking in" at this point, she may not be able to assimilate all the information that she wants or needs (Rubin, 1961). Having the father or another support person involved in the teaching will provide an information resource when the woman is ready to "take hold" (Rubin, 1961). Written information and instructions are an important supplement to the teaching done by the nurse or by media. One example of this is a collaborative project which provided each mother with a folder of information. This information was color coded according to general, self-care, and infant care. The packet was also divided into two sections—one for hospital reading and one for at-home reading (Hayes et al., 1981). Whatever the choice of method, the goal is to prepare parents to care for themselves and their infants.

Biophysical Knowledge Deficits—Self-care

General hygiene. Showering, hair washing, and perineal care are essentials of basic postpartum hygiene. The proper procedure for perineal care, especially wiping from front to back, ought to be emphasized. It may be helpful to include the psychological benefits of "looking good" for "feeling good."

Lochia and involution. Women may need to know the characteristics and duration of normal lochia and that perineal care is continued at home until cessation of the lochia. Warning signs of foul-smelling lochia or return of bright red lochia are included in the discussion. It is helpful to warn women that a dark brown lochia may occur with a sudden increase in activity. The involution process should be explained and the woman can be taught to palpate her fundus.

Incision. Care of the incision may be showering, sitz baths, perineal care, and positioning for an episiotomy. Women need to know that the episiotomy should be comfortable in about three weeks. If there have been lacerations or a hematoma, the discomfort may continue for a longer period of time. Analgesics may also be needed for a period of time at home. Part of the teaching process may be to help women look at their episiotomies if they so desire.

If the woman has had a cesarean delivery, care of the abdominal incision is included. Because the healing process can take up to two years (Bruno, 1979, pp. 668–670), women need to know what to expect during the different phases of wound healing. Teaching for home care includes reinforcing of instructions for activity. Usually lifting heavy objects is prohibited during the first two weeks (Bruno, 1979). Women will need to be shown how to pick up and hold their seven- or eight-pound newborns so that they do not stress the incision. Ambulation is encouraged to promote adequate blood flow to the area. Women may also need to know that the scar formation may be raised and purplish in color but that the color will diminish and the incision line will reduce in size (Bruno, 1979). Adequate nutrition is important for tissue healing and will be discussed in another section.

Gastrointestinal tract. Teaching in the hospital about exercise and diet which includes fresh fruit, vegetables, whole grains, and adequate fluid will prepare the woman to prevent constipation at home. If a bowel movement does not occur within two or three days, a cathartic or enema may be prescribed. Women should be cautioned about continued use of cathartics for bowel evacuation and stress should be placed on diet, exercise, and fluid (Hawkins & Higgins, 1981, Chap. 17).

Hemorrhoids can be a problem during the postpartum period as they can interfere with comfort and bowel functioning. In-hospital care that the woman can continue at home includes use of anesthetic sprays or ointments, ice packs, witch hazel compresses, sitz baths, and analgesics. Teaching includes information on how often and in what amounts to use these relief-producing methods. Again stress on diet and fluids to prevent constipation will aid the remission of hemorrhoidal discomfort (Hawkins & Higgins, 1981, Chap. 17).

Urinary tract. Prevention of urinary tract problems requires teaching which includes perineal care, relaxation and pelvic floor exercises (Kegel), and the need for fluids. If urinary retention occurs, catheterization may be required. This initially may be a straight catheter. Occasionally an indwelling catheter may have to be inserted for one to two days to allow for rest and healing to occur. Teaching about catheter care and management of a catheter is important. Rarely, a woman must go home with an indwelling catheter in place. When this occurs, the woman should be shown how to empty the collection bag and attach a leg collection bag. She must know how to do catheter care at home, including how to irrigate or remove the catheter if it should become blocked.

Breasts. Care of the breasts differs for the woman who is breast-feeding and for the woman who is not. The breast-feeding mother may already have some knowledge of breast care if she has done some preparation prenatally. Water washing only, avoiding soap, which is very drying, application of a lanolin-based cream, air drying after nursing, wearing a supportive bra, and changing bra pads when moist are basics of preventive care (Hawkins & Higgins, 1981, Chap. 17; Riordan & Countryman, 1980a). Engorgement in the nursing mother can be prevented by unrestricted nursing time (Riordan & Countryman, 1980a; Whitley, 1978). If engorgement occurs, women can be taught to apply warm, moist heat via towels or shower and to manually express milk if the infant has difficulty latching on to the nipple (Riordan & Countryman, 1980a). Prevention of sore, cracked nipples will be discussed in the section on breast-feeding. This type of information can be shared with women as part of a peer group class which serves for information transmission as well as for support (Grassley & Davis, 1978; Riordan & Countryman, 1980b).

The woman who is bottle feeding will experience engorgement about the third day after delivery. Use of a snug-fitting bra during the day and at night as well, application of ice packs, and analgesics will alleviate the discomfort. Women must be informed not to express milk or stimulate their nipples during this time to shut down the lactation cycle. Engorgement decreases significantly in a day or two, and the breasts return to near normal in two to three weeks. Women should also be warned that there may be some spontaneous leaking of milk during this time. Use of chemical lactation suppressants was discussed in Chapter 2. If the woman has received a lactation suppressant, she should still be prepared to manage rebound or delayed engorgement. If the lactation suppressant is to be continued at home, the woman should know how and when to take the medication as well as some of the side effects to observe. Mynick (1981) describes a self-medication program instituted on a postpartum unit, an ideal way of preparing women for taking medications at home. The woman who has chosen to breast-feed her infant needs special instructions about drugs excreted in breast milk. She should make clear to any physician under whose care she is prescribed medication that she is breast-feeding and should not use over-the-counter drugs without consulting a health care professional such as a pharmacist, nurse, or physician.

Teaching breast self-exam may not be ideal with a woman who has sore, tender breasts. The technique of breast self-exam and educational information regarding breast self-exam can be given to women and can be followed up at the postpartum visit or at breast-feeding support groups. Descriptive pamphlets can usually be obtained through the local chapter of The American Cancer Society. Women find 90 percent of breast cancers themselves (Townsend, 1980). Teaching and reinforcing preventive health measures is an important aspect of postpartum and self-care. Strelnick (1982) argues that postpartum is an opportune time to reinforce teaching about self-examination of breasts.

Nutrition. Closely tied with body image is the woman's concerns with losing her pregnancy weight. The restorative needs of the body, the demands of breast-feeding and infant care, and fatigue do not make postpartum a time for a calorie-restricted diet. Nutritional self-care needs may be as simple as instructing the breast-feeding mother that she needs 600 extra calories in her well-balanced diet (Riordan & Countryman, 1980a) or as complicated as teaching what constitutes a well-balanced diet of approximately 2,000 calories. This type of teaching can be done by instructional material, use of dietitian, and examples from hospital menu. Tissue healing requires vitamins A and C, protein, and minerals (Bruno, 1979). This may take on greater meaning to the woman who has had a cesarean delivery. Women may also need to know what resources are available for dietary counseling as follow-up or for supplemental food programs.

Activity/exercise/rest. The elation of the postpartum period can soon vanish in the dawn of interrupted sleep and demands of infant care. Preparing the woman for the first few weeks at home has components of home management that will allow the woman to rest when her infant is resting and to plan her activities, exercise time, and household chores. Ideally a support person will be available to take over those household chores so the woman can concentrate on herself and her infant. If no support person is available, community resources can be explored. Women should know how much activity including walking and stair climbing they should be doing. Some women may need more help in planning their activity if the physical layout of the home includes upstairs bedrooms and bath and downstairs living quarters.

Exercises can begin in the immediate postpartum. An example of exercise instructions that can be given to women during the postpartum hospital stay appears in an article by Ketter and Shelton (1983). These exercises include the pelvic tilt, also used in prenatal exercise sessions, the modified leg lift, a leg slide, and one designed to correct diastasis recti. An exercise program is helpful to restore the body to its prepregnant shape (or better) as well as improve the woman's sense of well-being. Deep breathing, abdominal, and pelvic floor exercises can be started in the hospital. These are beneficial to cesarean birth women as well as those who have had a vaginal delivery. The cesarean birth woman will also need help with splinting the incision. The abdominal and breathing exercises will help this woman to cope with postoperative gas pains and will increase pulmonary ventilation (Harris, 1980). An instruction sheet for exercises should be explained and given to women before discharge.

Contraception. Women must start thinking about the type of family planning method, if any, they will use before resuming intercourse. Resumption of sexual activity will be discussed later in this chapter. Even if the woman indicates that she is not planning to resume sexual activity, providing her with written information as a future reference may prevent a crisis. Women need to know that ovulation can occur before menses and during lactation. For non-breast-feeding women, foam and condoms are recommended during the six-week postpartum period. Some physicians will prescribe oral contraceptives to begin one to two weeks postpartum. Breast-feeding women use foam and condoms initially. Nurses should provide information and be prepared to answer questions about natural family planning methods, diaphragms, IUDs, foam and condoms, oral contraceptives, and sterilization.

Psychosocial Knowledge Deficits—Self-care

Anticipatory guidance is the key phrase for planning and intervention to meet the psychosocial learning needs of mothers and fathers. The areas that will be discussed in this section are body image, postpartum "blues," family integration, and sexual intimacy. As was stated earlier, the psychosocial needs are not separate entities from the biophysical needs but rather components of the whole picture of postpartum.

Body image. The reality that with delivery of the infant does not come the prepregnant figure soon descends on the postpartum woman. Gruis (1977) found the primary concern of women in postpartum was their figures. Self-esteem can certainly be tested in this society which emphasizes thinness, fad diets for rapid weight loss, health spas, and reducing salons. Restoration takes time. Teaching about exercises, nutrition, involution, and the time involved will help the woman cope and remain in precrisis. Words of encouragement that convey caring are important during this time.

Postpartum "blues." Women should be prepared to expect times when they may feel mildly depressed, tearful, anxious, and unable to concentrate. These are the signs of what is known as postpartum "blues" (Hawkins & Higgins, 1981, Chap. 17). There may be many contributing factors to this feeling. One is related to the fall in hormone levels of estrogen and progesterone. Another may be the demands of the infant, which lead to loss of sleep and interrupted sleep, perhaps the major factor in the "blues" (Hawkins & Higgins, 1981, Chap. 17). Having information about the "blues" may not prevent them from occurring but it may help the woman to know that this is normal and time restricted.

Family integration. One of the tasks of postpartum is attainment of a new role. Incorporating a new family member means changes in activity for all other family members until a new equilibrium is reached. Ventura (1982, p. 269) found in her study that parents who perceived their infants as having a more smiling, laughing temperament, and as children who cried less, used the following coping mechanisms: they were more religious, thankful, and content and tended to use coping strategies designed to maintain family integrity. Those parents who were depressed and anxious saw their babies as less soothable and more distressed and tended to use coping mechanisms such as social supports and self-development. Sheehan (1981) found the problems of postpartum to be with assumption of role and role conflict. Gruis (1977) found the second most important concern of women to be regulating the many demands of the husband, the house, and other children as well as the new infant. Postpartum nurses can provide support for this experience by implementing and/or leading peer support groups. Chesaro and Terek (1978) describe a support group which allows parents to verbalize their fears and anxieties about taking a new baby home. Sharing feelings decreases the isolation parents may sense. Family adjustments may also be enhanced by a follow-up phone call during the first week at home (Donaldson, 1977). Parents need to know what resources are available to them once they are home. These might be a public health nurse referral, a home visit by a follow-up clinician, or a visit by or to a nurse practitioner (Donaldson, 1981; Gruis, 1977; Marecki, 1979).

Sexual intimacy. Information given by the nurse to the woman and her husband or significant other may avert resumption of sexual activity from becoming a crisis of postpartum. The information given must be individualized to the woman's needs and must be based on fact. Masters and Johnson (1966) provide the basis for the physiologic differences of intercourse in the puerperium. There is a decrease in rapidity and response, and pelvic vasocongestion is delayed. The thinner walls of the vagina do not lubricate as well because of the decrease in estrogen. Lactating women may have leaking breasts during sexual activity and may continue to have vaginal dryness (Hames, 1980; Kyndely, 1978; Riordan & Countryman, 1980b). By three months postpartum, the nonpregnant response will be reestablished (Inglis, 1980; Kyndely, 1978). Most authors recommend resumption of intercourse when vaginal bleeding ceases and the episiotomy is comfortable (Hames, 1980; Inglis, 1980; Israel & Rubin, 1967; Kyndely, 1978). Hames (1980) found most couples resumed intercourse before six weeks. Counseling for this portion of postpartum self-care deals with the body changes that have occurred, positioning, use of water-soluble jelly for lubrication, and psychological readiness (Inglis, 1980). Breast-feeding women will need additional information about coping with leaking breasts by wearing a bra during sexual activity and about prolonged vaginal dryness. Women who have had a cesarean birth may need information on positions if the abdominal incision is tender (Harris, 1980). Contraceptive information as previously discussed should also be provided. Fatigue, fear, pain, and role conflict may interfere with satisfactory resumption of sexual intimacy. Kitzinger (1980) lists concepts of pollution (taboos), tiredness, depression, pain, breast-feeding, fear of contraception, and interruptions as some of the deterrents to sexual adjustment postpartum. Caregivers who are aware of these can help women and their partners to understand the array of stressors and find ways of coping that allow for time for intimacy. Some women feel guilty if they fail to abstain for six weeks as recommended by their physicians (Hames, 1980). An understanding partner and accurate knowledge play a large role in maintaining a precrisis equilibrium.

Biophysical Knowledge Deficits—Infant Care

Preventive intervention during postpartum incorporates information about caretaking. The role of mother consists of two components: an emotional one and a caretaking one (Ludington-Hoe, 1977). This section will consider the common caretaking activities that parents need experience with and information about during the hospital stay.

Bathing. Mothers, and fathers too, need information about sponge bathing and tub bathing an infant. Areas to stress are that bathing should be done in a warm, draft-free area, infants should not be left unattended, and infants are slippery when wet. Cleaning the face, creases, the umbilical cord until it falls off, the circumcision if appropriate, and the genital area are covered. Women may need to know about retracting the foreskin and cleaning an uncircumcised penis or that smegma between the female labia will gradually diminish. Parents should participate in the infant's care as much as they desire. Use of soaps, powder, and lotions should be discussed (Bishop, 1980, Chap. 11).

Diapering. Proper procedure for diapering, care and cleaning of diapers, and prevention and care of diaper rash should be addressed. Genital care, circumcision care, and umbilical cord care can all be reinforced with teaching about diapering. Nurses should have information about cost, availability, advantages and disadvantages of cloth versus disposable diapers, and of diaper cleaning service versus home cleaning. This is also a good time to teach or reinforce teaching about normal bowel evacuation as opposed to diarrhea or constipation.

Holding. Some parents need instruction on support of the infant's head and neck to prevent jerking. Cesarean birth women may need assistance in positioning their infants to avoid pressure on the mother's abdomen (Harris, 1980). All parents should be shown the football hold, which gives a sense of security when holding an infant.

Clothing. Overdressing infants is more common than underdressing. Parents should be told to dress their infants as they would themselves to be comfortable (Bishop, 1980, Chap. 11). Parents should be cautioned, however, about exposing the infant's delicate skin to direct sunlight. Also, in this energy-conscious age, many parents are keeping their home environments cooler in the winter months. Newborns have greater heat loss per unit of body weight than adults (Whaley & Wong, 1979, p. 257) and have more difficulty maintaining their body temperature. The average hospital nursery temperature should be 75°F, which adds to the stress on the newborn if the home environment is five or more degrees cooler. Informing parents about infant heat loss and proper clothing can prevent cold stress at home. Thus, the rule of thumb above might be modified to one more layer than for adults, taking into consideration cooler temperatures at home and energy conservation measures.

Temperature taking. Axillary and rectal temperature taking are of themselves anxiety-provoking skills for parents to learn. In addition to the procedure, parents need to know how to read a thermometer, what type of thermometer to buy, when to take a temperature, and what to report to the physician. Schiffman found in her investigation (1982, p. 274) that axillary temperature taking may be a practical method for taking infants' temperatures if the technique is used properly.

Feeding. Perhaps the most crucial aspect of caretaking is infant feeding. Emotional well-being of the parent and physical well-being of the infant depend on successful initiation and maintenance of feeding behavior. Bottle feeding women need information about how to hold the bottle so that the infant receives no air from the nipple, about average stomach content of the infant, and about how and when to burp as in Figure 6.1. Preparing for home care should include information concerning the increasing demands of the infant for food, assessing when the infant is full, and formula preparation. Nurses must be knowledgeable about the different types of glass and disposable bottles and the care of each and about the cost, availability, and preparation of the different types of formulas. Anticipatory guidance for the

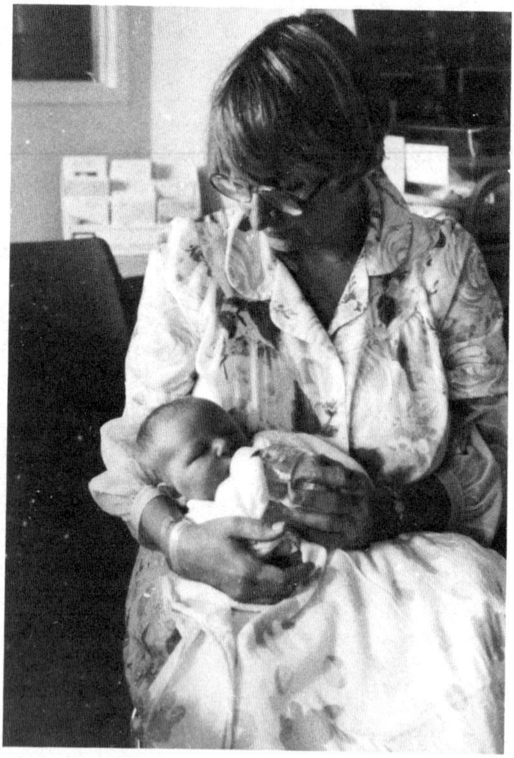

Figure 6.1 Bottle feeding. (Photograph by Bruce L. Beck.)

first few days at home consists of the woman's knowing how she is going to prepare the formula, sterilize the bottles, and use the correct nipple. Infants must have about two hours of sucking per day to satisfy their oral needs (Whaley & Wong, 1979, p. 286). For bottle-fed infants who feed approximately six times a day, 20 minutes of sucking should be allowed each feeding. Women may need to select the nipples which will allow this sucking time to occur. Emphasis should also be placed on the interaction time between woman and infant that feeding provides. Women should be encouraged to hold their infants during all feedings. Propping the bottle for feeding should be discouraged. This practice denies the infant social contact and places the infant at risk for aspiration and middle ear infection (Whaley & Wong, 1979, p. 286). Women may also need to address any feelings of guilt they may have about choosing to bottle feed their infants. Careful attention to the learning needs of the women who choose bottle feeding may eliminate one area of potential crisis.

The breast-feeding woman also needs support and information to initiate and maintain lactation and to meet the needs of her infant. Gulick found in her study (1982) that women who were successful at breast-feeding had higher scores on a breast-feeding information questionnaire, higher overall scores on breast-feeding information, and more sources of information about breast-feeding than those women who were unsuccessful. Thus, information about breast-feeding is very important to women who choose this method of feeding their infants. These women need guidance, assistance, and instructions about positioning themselves in bed or in a chair (as in Figure 6.2), about positioning the infant so that the infant can grasp one nipple and as much of the areola as possible, about offering both breasts at each feeding, about starting on alternate breasts, and about breaking the suction before removing the infant from the breast. Beske and Garvis found in their study of breast-feeding (1982, p. 177) that women identified encouragement and support, practical information, and help from hospital nurses as important to success. Time limits are no longer recommended for initial nursing times (Riordan & Countryman, 1980a; Whitley, 1978). These authors believe that time limits delay the peak of soreness until the woman is home where there are fewer resources for assistance and support. Time limits may also contribute to engorgement and may not allow the let-down reflex to occur (Riordan & Countryman, 1980a; Whitley, 1978). Breast care and nutritional care, as discussed earlier in this chapter, can be incorporated into teaching about breast-feeding.

Primary prevention for home care begins in the hospital with assessment and problem solving for inverted nipples, faulty position-

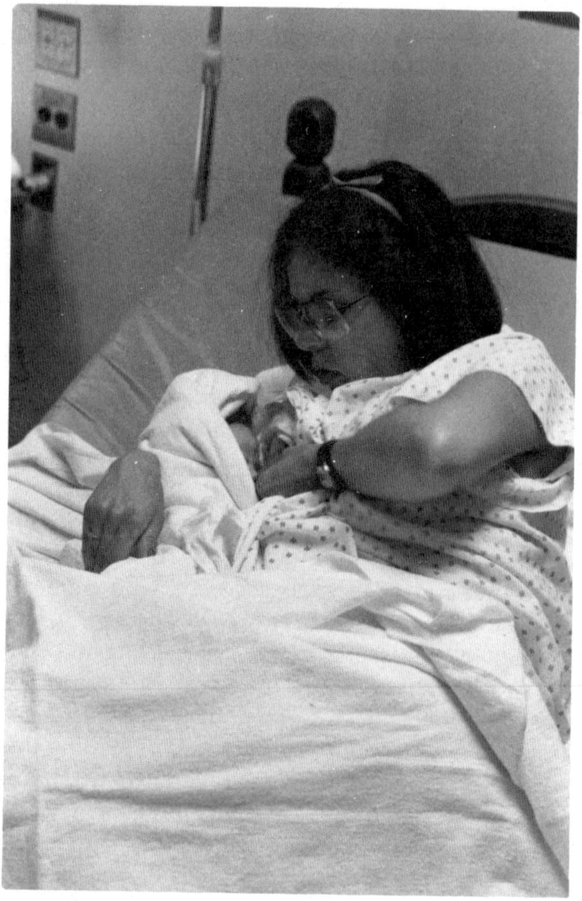

Figure 6.2 Breast-feeding. (Photograph by Richard Ramos.)

ing, inappropriate suckling problems, and sore nipples. Women should be given interventions they can carry out if these problems are identified. Different positions for feeding can be tried in the hospital. Instruction for alterations in breast-feeding to accommodate sore nipples can also be distributed. Women also need to know some basic expectations for their breast-feeding infants. Breast-feeding infants nurse 8 to 12 times a day and their soft to liquid stools may occur with each feeding (Riordan & Countryman, 1980b). On the other hand, some breast-fed infants stool as infrequently as every two days or so and their bowel movements are soft. Women's fears about underfeeding their infants can be allayed with knowledge that a baby whose color and skin tone are good, who nurses every two to three hours, who has six to eight wet diapers a day, and who seems generally well is probably receiving adequate nutrition (Riordan & Countryman, 1980b).

Women must be prepared for the demands that breast-feeding will place on them during the first few weeks at home. Fatigue can easily result if the woman is not prepared to rest when possible and if the mother does not have supports available to assist with or do the household tasks. Women should also be told of resources available to them at home. These may include peer support groups such as La Leche League, a public health nurse, another empathetic nurse in her community, or the nurse practitioner or pediatrician. Women should also be prepared for the increased sexual feelings they may have while breast-feeding and for the let-down reflex occurring when they think about their infants, and during intercourse. Preliminary information about expressing and storing milk can be given in the hospital. The support and guidance that women receive from nurses in the hospital can spell the difference between equilibrium and crisis.

Psychosocial Knowledge Deficits—Infant Care

The accommodation of a new family member is a very important process. This process begins in the hospital. Attachment behaviors described in Chapter 5 can be observed during the hospital portion of the puerperium. Infant behaviors can be identified using tools described in Chapter 5. These tools as well as performing newborn physical assessment with the parents present can be used to introduce their infant to them. Questions about the infant's appearance can be answered. Infant reflexes and how to elicit and utilize them can be demonstrated as in Figure 6.3. Riesch (1979) showed that women expected and observed behaviors in their infants but did not perceive these behaviors as having a purpose, that of social interaction. Showing parents that these and other behaviors are the infant's way of communicating or responding to them can help parents to see the individuality of their infant and to respond to the interaction cues that their infant is emitting. Parents can also plan the home environment to enhance their infant's development by placing objects eight inches away from the infant, using colors and patterns, changing mobiles, and providing happy human faces (Whaley & Wong, 1979, p. 279). Explanations about states of sleep and crying activity have implications for parenting. This helps parents determine when and if to stimulate the infant, when to pick the infant up from the crib, and what stimuli decrease crying (Whaley & Wong, 1979, p. 278). Infants need time to develop circadian rhythms that are synchronized with the adult family's rhythms. This may take

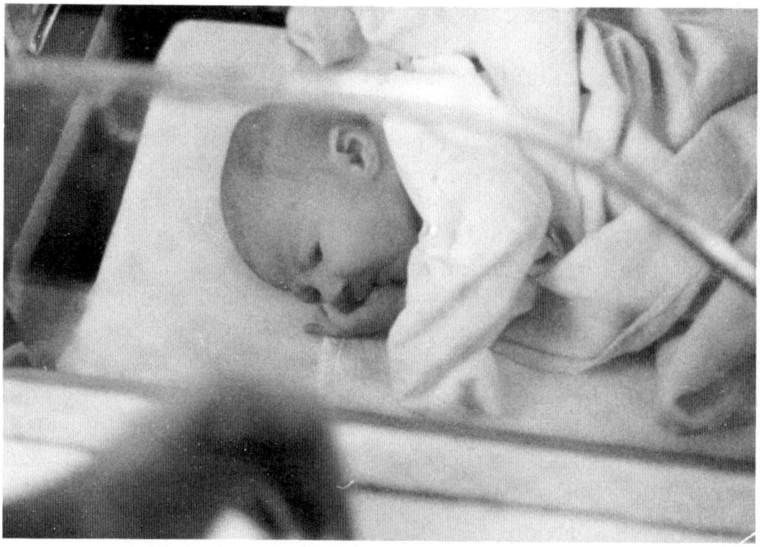

Figure 6.3 Observing normal infant behavior. (Photograph by Louise Baduski.)

weeks and some children perhaps are never synchronized with their parents (Deters, 1980). It is felt that the close interaction between mother and infant helps adult rhythms to develop in the infant (Deters, 1980).

Other members of the family have needs relating to acceptance of the new member. Parents may need guidance on facilitating attachment with siblings and dealing with sibling rivalry. Many institutions are now permitting sibling visitation. Parents may also need guidance on incorporating grandparents into family structure. Parents' coping mechanisms may need to be augmented to deal with new situations.

Identification and Utilization of Community Resources

Ideally, the nurse who provides postpartum care for women and their infants in the postpartum setting will be knowledgeable about community resources and work in close collaboration with community health nurses in the local visiting nurse service, the county or city health department, or well child services. A resource guide for community services and agencies should be available on the postpartum unit if at all possible. Referral forms for the local health department or visiting nurse service should be available and nurses instructed on how to make a referral when first employed.

Resources for women and their families within the local community might include the following: family planning clinics, including those in local hospitals (if any) as well as those sponsored by organizations such as Planned Parenthood League; well baby services under the auspices of the visiting nurse service for the community or the local health department or outpatient services of a hospital; WIC programs for nutrition supplementation; the cooperative extension services of the Department of Agriculture (especially in rural areas); March of Dimes chapters for information for families with a child with a birth defect; services for handicapped children under state health programs; parents groups run under the aegis of the childbirth education group in the community, the local "Y," churches, or synagogues; La Leche League; and parent support groups such as for parents of twins. Sources of information include the telephone directory (blue pages for municipal services); published guides to state or local health and welfare services (many communities and states have these); local, county, or state health departments; health care institutions and agencies within the community; and voluntary groups such as the Junior League.

Summary

Inpatient postpartum is a time of potential crisis. It is also a time of primary prevention for future hazardous events. The teaching the nurse does during this short time is very valuable in assisting the woman to balance her needs and her infant's needs. There are many tasks to be accomplished during the puerperium and sometimes little energy to tackle them. The nurse is in a pivotal position to support the woman through this experience by being attentive to readiness to learn, by teaching what parents want to know, and by providing resources for the woman post-hospitalization. These interventions will be the balancing factors needed to maintain equilibrium: an accurate perception of the event, support systems, and resources for coping augmentation.

References

Beske, J., & Garvis, M. S. Important factors in breast-feeding success. *The American Journal of Maternal Child Nursing*, 1982, *7*(3), 174–179.

Bishop, B. *The maternity cycle: One nurse's reflections*. Philadelphia: F. A. Davis, 1980.

Bruno, P. The nature of wound healing. *Nursing Clinics of North America*, 1979, *14*, 667–682.

Campbell, S., & Smith, J. Postpartum: Assessment guide. *American Journal of Nursing*, 1977, *77*, 1179.

Chesaro, F. J., & Terek, R. E. Pillow talk—a comfort for new mothers. *The American Journal of Maternal Child Nursing*, 1978, *3*, 183–184.

Cronenwett, L. R., & Kunst-Wilson, W. Stress, social support, and the transition to fatherhood. *Nursing Research*, 1981, *30*, 196–201.

Croog, E. H., & Zigrossi, S. T. Parenting luncheons on the postpartum unit. *The American Journal of Maternal Child Nursing*, 1983, *8*(4), 277–279.

Deters, G. E. Circadian rhythm phenomenon. *The American Journal of Maternal Child Nursing*, 1980, *5*, 249–251.

Donaldson, N. E. Fourth trimester follow-up. *American Journal of Nursing*, 1977, *77*, 1176–1178.

Donaldson, N. E. The postpartum follow-up nurse clinician. *Journal of Obstetric, Gynecologic, and Neonatal Nursing*, 1981, *10*, 249–254.

Grassley, J. G., & Davis, K. Common concerns of mothers who breast feed. *The American Journal of Maternal Child Nursing*, 1978, *3*, 347–351.

Greenberg, M., & Morris, N. Engrossment: The newborn's impact upon the father. *American Journal of Orthopsychiatry*, 1974, *44*, 520–531.

Gruis, M. Beyond maternity: Postpartum concerns of mothers. *The American Journal of Maternal Child Nursing*, 1977, *2*, 182–188.

Gulick, E. E. Informational correlates of successful breast-feeding. *The American Journal of Maternal Child Nursing*, 1982, *7*(6), 370–375.

Hames, C. T. Sexual needs and interests of postpartum couples. *Journal of Obstetric, Gynecologic, and Neonatal Nursing*, 1980, *9*, 313–315.

Harris, J. K. Self-care is possible after cesarean delivery. *Nursing Clinics of North America*, 1980, *15*, 191–204.

Hawkins, J. W., & Higgins, L. P. *Maternity and gynecologic nursing: Women's health care*. Philadelphia: Lippincott, 1981.

Hayes, E. R., Miner, N., Orne, R., White, M. F., & Gentes, N. W. Meeting the health teaching needs of new and expanding families in Rockville. University of Connecticut, Rockville General Hospital, Rockville Public Health Nursing Association. Regional Project to Improving Nursing Services and Nursing Education in Maternal and Child Health Care. Final Report—Group III, May 1981. Storrs: University of Connecticut School of Nursing.

Howley, C. The older primipara. Implications for nurses. *Journal of Obstetric, Gynecologic, and Neonatal Nursing*, 1981, *10*, 182–185.

Inglis, T. Postpartum sexuality. *Journal of Obstetric, Gynecologic, and Neonatal Nursing*, 1980, *9*, 298–300.

Israel, S. L., & Rubin, I. *Sexual relations during pregnancy and the post-delivery period* (Study Guide No. 6). New York: Sex Information and Education Council of the United States, 1967.

Ketter, D. E., & Shelton, B. J. In-hospital exercises for the postpartal woman. *The American Journal of Maternal Child Nursing*, 1983, *8*(2), 120–124.

Kitzinger, S. *Sex after the baby comes*. Seattle, Wash.: Pennypress, 1980.

Knowles, M. S. *The modern practice of adult education*. New York: Association Press, 1970.
Kyndely, K. The sexuality of women in pregnancy and postpartum: A review. *Journal of Obstetric, Gynecologic, and Neonatal Nursing*, 1978, *7*, 28–32.
Ludington-Hoe, S. M. Postpartum: Development of maternicity. *American Journal of Nursing*, 1977, *77*, 1171–1174.
Marecki, M. P. Postpartum follow-up goals and assessment. *Journal of Obstetric, Gynecologic, and Neonatal Nursing*, 1979, *8*, 214–218.
Masters, W. H., & Johnson, V. E. *Human sexual response*. Boston: Little, Brown, 1966.
Mynick, A. Instituting a postpartum self-medication program. *The American Journal of Maternal Child Nursing*, 1981, *6*(6), 422–424.
Riesch, S. Enhancement of mother-infant social interaction. *Journal of Obstetric, Gynecologic, and Neonatal Nursing*, 1979, *8*, 242–246.
Riordan, J., & Countryman, B. A. Basics of breast feeding. Part IV: Preparation for breast feeding and early optimal functioning. *Journal of Obstetric, Gynecologic, and Neonatal Nursing*, 1980, *9*, 277–283. (a)
Riordan, J., & Countryman, B. A. Basics of breast feeding. Part V: Self-care for continued breast feeding. *Journal of Obstetric, Gynecologic, and Neonatal Nursing*, 1980, *9*, 357–361. (b)
Riordan, J., & Countryman, B. A. Basics of breast feeding. Part VI: Some breast feeding problems and solutions. *Journal of Obstetric, Gynecologic, and Neonatal Nursing*, 1980, *9*, 361–366. (c)
Rubin, R. Puerperal change. *Nursing Outlook*, 1961, *9*, 753–755.
Rubin, R. Maternity nursing stops too soon. *American Journal of Nursing*, 1975, *75*, 1680–1684.
Schiffman, R. F. Temperature monitoring in the neonate: A comparison of axillary and rectal temperatures. *Nursing Research*, 1982, *31*(5), 274–277.
Schmidt, J. Using a teaching guide for better postpartum and infant care. *Journal of Obstetric, Gynecologic, and Neonatal Nursing*, 1978, *7*(3), 23–26.
Sheehan, F. Assessing postpartum adjustment. A pilot study. *Journal of Obstetric, Gynecologic, and Neonatal Nursing*, 1981, *10*, 19–23.
Strelnick, E. G. Postpartum care: An opportunity to reinforce breast self-examination. *The American Journal of Maternal Child Nursing*, 1982, *7*(4), 249–252.
Sumner, G., & Fritsch, J. Postnatal parental concerns: The first six weeks of life. *Journal of Obstetric, Gynecologic, and Neonatal Nursing*, 1977, *6*(3), 27–32.
Taubenheim, A. M. Paternal-infant bonding in the first-time father. *Journal of Obstetric, Gynecologic, and Neonatal Nursing*, 1981, *10*, 261–264.
Townsend, C. B., Jr. Breast lumps. *Clinical Symposia*, 1980, *32*(2), 1–32.
Ventura, J. N. Parent coping behaviors, parent functioning, and infant temperament characteristics. *Nursing Research*, 1982, *31*(5), 269–273.
Whaley, L. F., & Wong, D. L. *Nursing care of infants and children*. St. Louis: C. V. Mosby, 1979.
Whitley, N. Preparation for breast feeding. A one-year follow-up of 34 nursing mothers. *Journal of Obstetric, Gynecologic, and Neonatal Nursing*, 1978, *7*(3), 44–48.

7

Assessment of High-risk Factors in Parenting

Introduction

As pregnancy nears completion, the parents' thoughts focus in on the events that will surround the infant's birth. For many parents, the thought (fear) of giving birth to an infant with health problems becomes more predominant than in previous months of the pregnancy. Rubin (1970) has identified emotional adaptations that take place during the three trimesters of pregnancy. During the third trimester there is a protective feeling toward the infant and a readiness to deliver and view a healthy baby. When parents imagine what the child will be like, they often anticipate the "picture-book" baby, attractive, bright, and well-developed.They envision periods of growth and sharing with the new child that will provide much joy and enrichment in their lives. Howell (1973) states further that parents also enjoy the thought of reproducing themselves by giving birth to a healthy, beautiful child.

Stress is produced in the parents when their anticipation of the healthy imagined child is marred by their fear of delivering a child that is displaying a defect or health problem. Parents are allowed very little opportunity to express this fear. When brought to the surface, the parents' concern is quickly suppressed by statements such as: "Don't say that!" "How foolish to think that way." "That's silly." "The baby will be fine so don't talk about any problem." Childbirth groups can provide support to the parents passing through this stress period in pregnancy by encouraging the sharing of feelings surrounding this emotional issue.

It is apparent that although most parents are aware of the possibility of a complication occurring with their unborn child, they are not envisioning the child as a high-risk infant. Consequently, the birth of a high-risk infant leaves the parents in a crisis state. The parents suffer the loss of the healthy, imagined child and face the unpredictable future with the real child. The purpose of this chapter is to discuss the parents' response to the child's birth and the role of the nurse in support and intervention.

Assessment for Risk Factors

In some instances, it is possible to predict the birth of a high-risk infant, as illustrated in Table 7.1. Klaus and Farnaroff (1979) have described high-risk factors contributing to perinatal mortality and morbidity in infants. The value of an accurate nursing history is evident in reviewing high-risk factors. Family history in relation to serious hereditary and familial abnormalities, significant congenital anomalies, and socioeconomic problems may provide the individual with valuable preconception information in decision making regarding pregnancy. Maternal history including a thorough medical/surgical/obstetrical review may provide clues as to the possibilities of complications in the newborn. The prenatal course may reveal additional or unanticipated factors that can lead to a high-risk situation at birth. A high-risk situation may occur only during labor or following delivery.

In order to assess the newborn at birth, the nurse initially may obtain some indication of the status of the infant by obtaining the Apgar score at one and five minutes. A more comprehensive tool used to determine gestational age and neurological functioning was developed by Dubowitz, Dubowitz, and Goldberg (1970) and appears in Tables 7.2 and 7.3 and Figure 7.1.

The need for frequent assessment of any high-risk infant has usually led to the newborn being placed in the special care unit after delivery. Parents often have difficulty in accepting and understanding the prophylactic need to place their infant in a special care nursery if the infant is not exhibiting distress or difficulties of any nature. The nurse needs to reinforce the importance of close observation of the high-risk infant when providing support to the parents.

Table 7.1 High-risk Factors Contributing to Perinatal Mortality and Morbidity in Infants

PRECONCEPTION--An awareness of the risk factor will place the decision about further procreation squarely with the parents

<u>Family History</u>

Serious hereditary and familial abnormalities--cystic fibrosis, osteogenesis imperfecta, Down's syndrome

Significant congenital anomalies involving the central nervous system, heart, or skeletal system

Blood dyscrasias--sickle cell disease

Socioeconomic problems--poor nutrition, unmarried and adolescent mother, ethnic background, medical indigency

<u>Maternal History</u>

Metabolic disease in the mother
- Endocrine--thyroid disease
- Amino acid--phenylketonuria
- Carbohydrate--diabetes
- Mucopolysaccharidoses

History of reproductive failures
- Miscarriage
- Toxemia of pregnancy
- Prolonged period of infertility
- Size of infant--history of previous premature or "small-for-dates" births

Anemia
- Sickle cell disease
- Thrombocytopenic purpura
- Hematocrit below 32 percent

Height and weight
- Height under 60 inches
- Prepregnant weight of less than 20 percent under or over the standards for weight and height
- Smoking

<u>Obstetrical Factors</u>

Maternal age
- Elderly primipara (over 35 years)
- Age over 30 years after short interpregnancy periods
- Age under 16 years

Excessive multiparity (over 5), especially when the mother is over 35 years of age

Table 7.1 (Continued)

Obstetric complications, past or present
- Blood group incompatibility
- Toxemia of pregnancy
- Placental separation
- Polyhydramnios or oligohydramnios

Paternal age over 40

PRENATAL--A number of factors occurring during pregnancy will alert the physician to the possibility of complications in the fetus, or ultimately in the newborn infant

Medical factors

Maternal infection

Maternal medications

Maternal drug addiction--narcotics, barbiturates, amphetamines, LSD

Socioeconomic problems
- Poor nutrition
- Illegitimacy
- Absence of father
- Lack of prenatal care--long-delayed or absent

Stressful events
- Severe emotional tension
- Hyperemesis gravidarum
- Operations for surgical problems during pregnancy, especially under general anesthesia--appendicitis, cholecystitis, intestinal obstruction, pelvic neoplasm
- Critical accidents

Radiation

Cardiovascular disease
- Congenital heart disease
- Hypertension

Renal disease

Diabetes

Myasthenia gravis

Intercurrent chronic disease--pyelonephritis, malignancy

(*continued*)

Table 7.1 (Continued)

Obstetrical Factors

Abnormal presentation--breech, transverse, unengaged presenting part at term

Fetus that fails to gain normally or is disparate in size from that expected

Fetus over 42 weeks' gestation

Multiple birth

Toxemia of pregnancy (eclampsia and preeclampsia)

Fetal heart aberrations

Rh sensitization

Hemorrhagic complications--abruptio placentae, placenta previa, rupture of marginal sinus

Uterine rupture

Indication for caesarean section

Polyhydramnios or oligohydramnios

Cord prolapse

NATAL--A high-risk situation may occur only during labor or following delivery; hence the importance of constant observation and monitoring during labor and delivery and postnatally

Maternal or Fetal Conditions During Labor

Fever, other signs of infection

Premature onset of labor

Premature rupture of membranes

Fetal distress (tachycardia, bradycardia, meconium staining of amniotic fluid)

Fetal scalp blood showing asphyxia (pH 7.2 or lower)

Prolonged labor

Precipitous delivery

Complicated delivery

Caesarean section

Table 7.1 (Continued)

Tight nuchal cord

Cord prolapse

Uterine rupture

Abruptio placentae

Heavy maternal sedation and/or anesthesia

Infant at Birth

Congenital anomalies (choanal atresia, micrognathia with cleft palate, diaphragmatic hernia, tracheoesophageal fistula, cardiovascular anomalies,imperforate anus)

Single umbilical artery

Breech or other abnormal delivery

Meconium staining

Low Apgar score, especially at five minutes

Placental abnormality (massive infarction, amnionitis, amnion nodosum)

Multiple birth

Prematurity

Disproportion between weight or length and gestational age

Depression

Birth trauma

Abnormal respiration

Sepsis

Severe blood loss

Severe hemolytic disease

POSTNATAL

Infant in the Nursery

Abnormal respiration

Apneic episodes

(continued)

Table 7.1 (Continued)

Tremors
Convulsions
Vomiting
Abdominal distention
Failure to pass meconium (24 hours)
Melena
Pallor
Petechiae
Jaundice--especially in first 24 hours
Thermal instability
Lethargy
Failure to void
Failure to regain birth weight by 10 days of age

Used with permission. From Klaus, M. H., & Farnaroff, A. A., Care of the High-Risk Newborn, 2nd ed., Philadelphia: W. B. Saunders Co., 1979.

Parents' Response to the Birth of a High-risk Infant

Theoretical Concepts

Parents experience a tremendous outpouring of emotional responses to the birth of a high-risk infant, often ranging from overwhelming loss and grief to guilt and anger. Solnit and Stark (1961) have described the mother's reaction to the birth of a defective child as similar in aspects to the mourning of the death of a child. It is important to understand that a perceived loss is just as important as a real loss. For example, an infant exhibiting no distress or problem may be sent to the special care nursery for a short observational period. The parents may clearly perceive their child as being critically ill by virtue of his or her placement in a high-risk setting. The loss is just as real, even though the person has created it, and the parents will experience emotional response to the loss.

It is known that grief is a normal response to a loss. Lindemann (1944) has concluded that normal grief is a definite syndrome. It includes:

1. Somatic distress with tightness of the throat, choking, shortness of breath, need for sighing, and an empty feeling in the abdomen, lack of muscular power, and an intense subjective distress described as tension or mental pain.
2. Preoccupation with the image of the deceased.
3. Feelings of guilt and preoccupation with one's negligence or minor omissions.
4. Feelings of hostility toward others.
5. Breakdown of normal patterns of conduct.

The family who gives birth to a high-risk infant experiences grief. *Grief work* is the term often used to indicate the internal process that a person undergoes in accomplishing a resolution to the loss. Grief is a painful process that the person must pass through in order to overcome the loss. Grief usually has a predictable path. Kübler-Ross (1969) has described common reactions in the grief process: denial and isolation; anger; bargaining; depression; and acceptance. The process is normally limited to several months' duration. In many cultures it is expected that grief will be expressed in a prescribed way. In the American culture the work of grieving is often left only partially done, resulting in delayed grief reactions appearing at a later time. It is important to realize that grief is a personal feeling and people will react differently. Reactions are varied and often contradictory. People may move through the stages of grief at a different pace. This may be difficult for family members to understand. Often the person who contains his grief within, not exhibiting observable responses to the loss, may be considered to be coping. Inwardly, however, he or she may be experiencing great turmoil. Too often society expects the man particularly to be strong and resolve the loss quickly.

The family who gives birth to a high-risk infant needs help in handling the stressful event and restoring equilibrium. According to Caplan (1964, p. 38), humans are constantly confronted with the need to problem-solve in order to maintain equilibrium. When confronted with an imbalance between a difficult problem and individual available coping

Table 7.2 Scoring System of External Physical Characteristics*

External Sign	Score				
	0	1	2	3	4
Edema	Obvious edema of hands and feet; pitting over tibia	No obvious edema of hands and feet; pitting over tibia	No edema		
Skin texture	Very thin, gelatinous	Thin and smooth	Smooth; medium thickness; rash or superficial peeling	Slight thickening. Superficial cracking and peeling, especially of hands and feet	Thick and parchment-like; superficial or deep cracking
Skin color	Dark red	Uniformly pink	Pale pink; variable over body	Pale; only pink over ears, lips, palms, or soles	
Skin opacity (trunk)	Numerous veins and venules clearly seen, especially abdomen	Veins and tributaries seen	A few large vessels clearly seen over abdomen	A few large vessels seen indistinctly over abdomen	No blood vessels seen
Lanugo (over back)	No lanugo	Abundant; long and thick over whole back	Hair thinning especially over lower back	Small amount of lanugo and bald areas	At least half of back devoid of lanugo

Table 7.2 (Continued)

External Sign	Score 0	1	2	3	4
Plantar creases	No skin creases	Faint red marks over anterior half of sole	Definite red marks marks over > anterior half; indentations over > anterior 1/3	Indentations over > anterior 1/3	Definite deep indentations over > anterior 1/3
Nipple formation	Nipple barely visible; no areola	Nipple well defined; areola smooth and flat, diameter < 0.75 cm	Areola stippled, edge not raised, diameter < 0.75 cm	Areola stippled, edge raised, diameter < 0.75 cm	
Breast size	No breast tissue palpable	Breast tissue on one or both sides, < 0.5 cm diameter	Breast tissue both sides; one or both 0.5 to 1.0 cm	Breast tissue both sides; one or both > 1 cm	
Ear form	Pinna flat and shapeless, little or no incurving of edge	Incurving part of edge of pinna	Partial incurving whole of upper pinna	Well-defined incurving whole of upper pinna	
Ear firmness	Pinna soft, easily folded, no recoil	Pinna soft easily folded, slow recoil	Cartilage to edge of pinna but soft in places, ready recoil	Pinna firm, cartilage to edge; instant recoil	

Table 7.2 (Continued)

External Sign	Score				
	0	1	2	3	4
Genitals: Male	Neither testis in scrotum	At least one testis high in scrotum	At least one testis right down		
Genitals: Female (with hips 1/2 abducted)	Labia majora widely separated, labia minora protruding	Labia majora almost cover labia minora	Labia majora completely cover labia minora		

Used with permission. Dubowitz, L., Dubowitz, V., & Goldberg, C. Clinical Assessment of Gestational Age in the Newborn Infant. Journal of Pediatrics, 77(1), 1970.

If score differs on two sides, take the mean.

abilities, a crisis may occur. Caplan (1964, pp. 40–41) described four developmental phases in a crisis:

1. There is an initial rise in tension as habitual problem-solving techniques are tried.
2. There is a lack of success in coping as the stimulus continues and more discomfort is felt.
3. A further increase in tension acts as a powerful internal stimulus and mobilizes internal and external resources. In this stage, emergency problem-solving mechanisms are tried. The problem may be redefined or there may be resignation and the giving up of certain aspects of the goal as unattainable.
4. If the problem continues and can be neither solved nor avoided, tension increases and a major disorganization occurs.

Figure 7.2 displays the effect of balancing factors when a person is faced with a stressful situation. In order to regain equilibrium, certain balancing factors must be present. When one or more balancing factors are absent, a crisis may develop (Aguilera & Messick, 1974, p. 61). Figure 7.3 can be utilized after assessing the following:

Case Study: Birth of a Premature Infant

Elizabeth and Jack H. were a healthy young couple, both in their mid-20s, who had been married for three years. They had been joyfully awaiting the birth of their first child. They attended childbirth classes, and Elizabeth had decided to breast-feed the baby. Elizabeth went into premature labor at seven months gestation. Up to this point her pregnancy had been uncomplicated and her overall health status excellent. The male baby, delivered at two and one-half pounds, was immediately transported to the regional neonatal center accompanied by Jack.

After a brief recovery period in the delivery area, Elizabeth was transferred to the postpartum unit. During the initial admission history to the unit, Elizabeth was very quiet. When questioned regarding the baby, Elizabeth began to cry and stated, "I can't believe this has happened. I took such good care of myself. What did I do wrong?"

Intervention. The nurse caring for Elizabeth needs to realize that she is in a state of mourning and experiencing disbelief and guilt at the premature birth of her baby. It is vital that Elizabeth be encouraged to

Table 7.3 Techniques of Neurological Assessment*

Posture

With the infant supine and quiet, score as follows:

arms and legs extended	= 0
slight or moderate flexion of hips and knees	= 1
moderate to strong flexion of hips and knees	= 2
legs flexed and abducted, arms slightly flexed	= 3
full flexion of arms and legs	= 4

Square Window

Flex the hand at the wrist. Exert pressure sufficient to get as much flexion as possible. The angle between the hypothenar eminence and the anterior aspect of the forearm is measured and scored according to Figure 7.1. Do not rotate the wrist.

Ankle Dorsiflexion

Flex the foot at the ankle with sufficient pressure to get maximum change. The angle between the dorsum of the foot and the anterior aspect of the leg is measured and scored as in Figure 7.1.

Arm Recoil

With the infant supine, fully flex the forearm for five seconds, then fully extend by pulling the hands and release. Score the reaction according to:

remain extended or random movements	= 0
incomplete or partial flexion	= 1

Popliteal Angle

With the infant supine and the pelvis flat on the examining surface, the leg is flexed on the thigh and the thigh fully flexed with the use of one hand. With the other hand the leg is then extended and the angle attained scored as in Figure 7.1.

Heel-to-Ear Maneuver

With the infant supine, hold the infant's foot with one hand and move it as near to the head as possible without forcing it. Keep the pelvis flat on the examining surface. Score as in Figure 7.1.

Scarf Sign

With the infant supine, take the infant's hand and draw it across the neck and as far across the opposite shoulder as possible. Assistance to the elbow is permissible by lifting it across the body. Score according to the location of the elbow:

elbow reaches the opposite anterior axillary line	= 0
elbow between opposite anterior axillary line and midline of thorax	= 1
elbow at midline of thorax	= 2
elbow does not reach midline of thorax	= 3

Head Lag

With the infant supine, grasp each forearm just proximal to the wrist and pull gently so as to bring the infant to a sitting position. Score according to the relationship of the head to the trunk during the maneuver:

Table 7.3 (Continued)

brisk return to full flexion = 2

Leg Recoil

With the infant supine, the hips and knees are fully flexed for five seconds, then extended by traction on the feet and released. Score the reaction according to:

no response or slight flexion = 0

partial flexion = 1

full flexion (less than 90^0 at knees and hips) = 2

no evidence of head support = 0

some evidence of head support = 1

maintains head in the same anteroposterior plane as the body = 2

tends to hold the head forward = 3

Ventral Suspension

With the infant prone and the chest resting on the examiner's palm, lift the infant off the examining surface and score according to the posture shown in Figure 7.1.

Used with permission. Dubowitz, L., Dubowitz, V., & Goldberg, C. Clinical Assessment of Gestational Age in the Newborn Infant. Journal of Pediatrics, 77(1), 1970.

*According to Dubowitz et al. from Amiel-Tison. To be used in conjunction with Figure 7.1.

verbalize her fears and anxieties. Although false reassurances and promises of the baby's recovery are inappropriate, it is important to convey as much hope and optimism as is allowable for the baby's condition. Elizabeth needs support in understanding that she did not "do anything wrong" to bring about premature labor. Parents of a high-risk infant frequently blame themselves, each other, or a specific upsetting event as the cause of the premature birth. Elizabeth will need to recognize her loss of the "imagined, healthy child" as she begins dealing with her newborn son.

Four tasks have been delineated for a woman to accomplish following the birth of a premature baby:

1. She must realize that she may lose the baby.
2. She must acknowledge failure in her maternal function to deliver a full-term baby.
3. After separation from the infant due to its prolonged

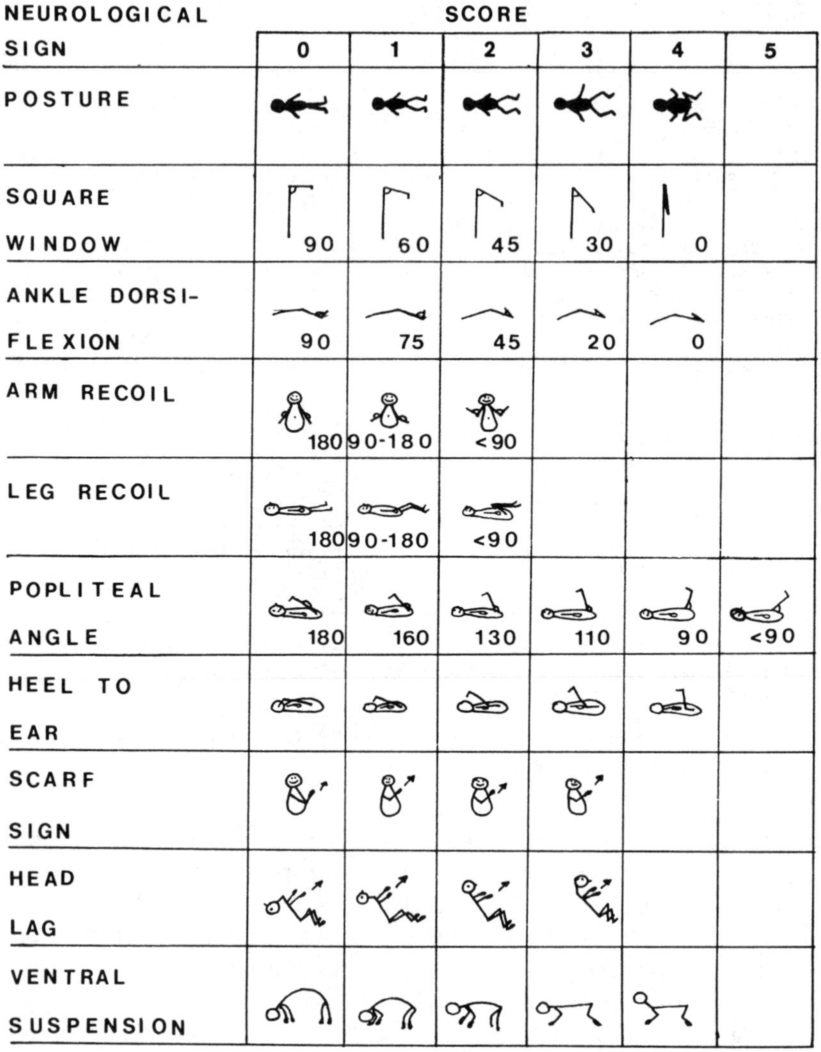

Figure 7.1 Neurological criteria for assessment of gestational age. (Used with permission from Dubowitz, L. M. S., Dubowitz, V., & Goldberg, C. "Clinical Assessment of Gestational Age in the Newborn Infant." *Journal of Pediatrics,* 1970, *77*(1), pp. 1–10.)

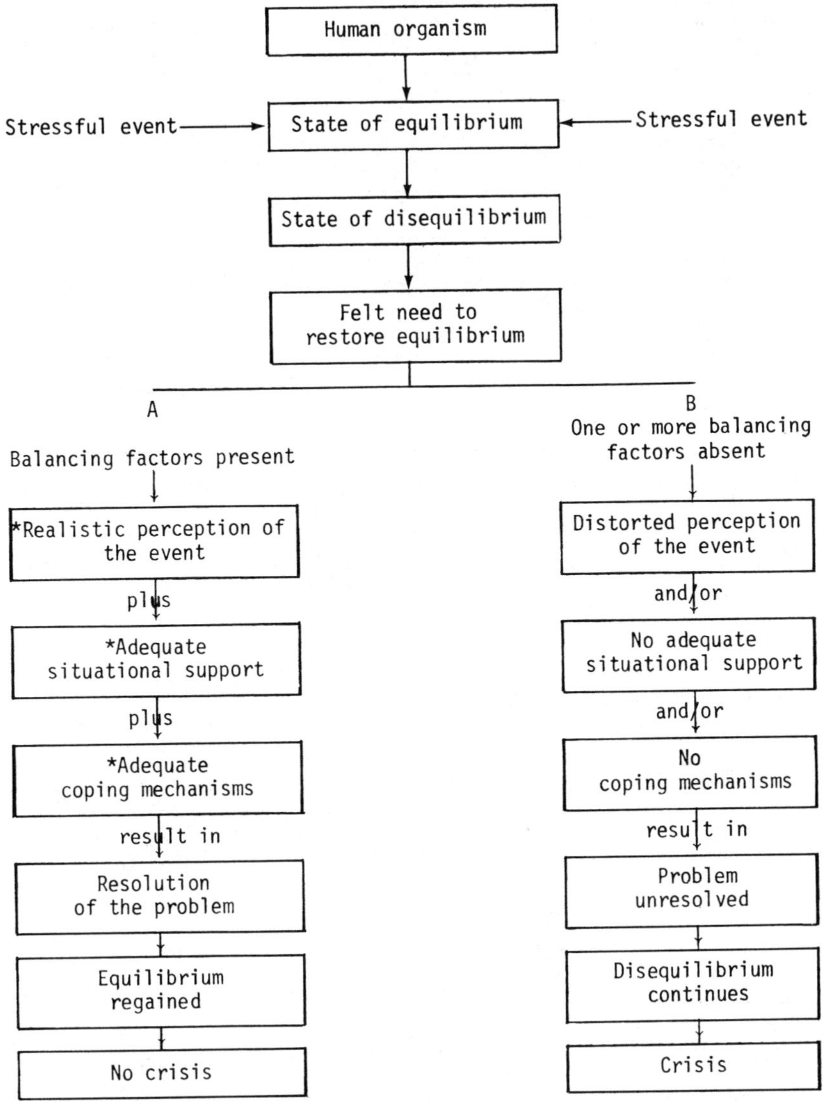

*Balancing factors.

Figure 7.2 Paradigm: Effect of balancing factors in a stressful event. (Used with permission. From Aguilera, Donna C., & Messick, Janice M. *Crisis Intervention*, 4th ed. St. Louis, The C. V. Mosby Co., 1982.)

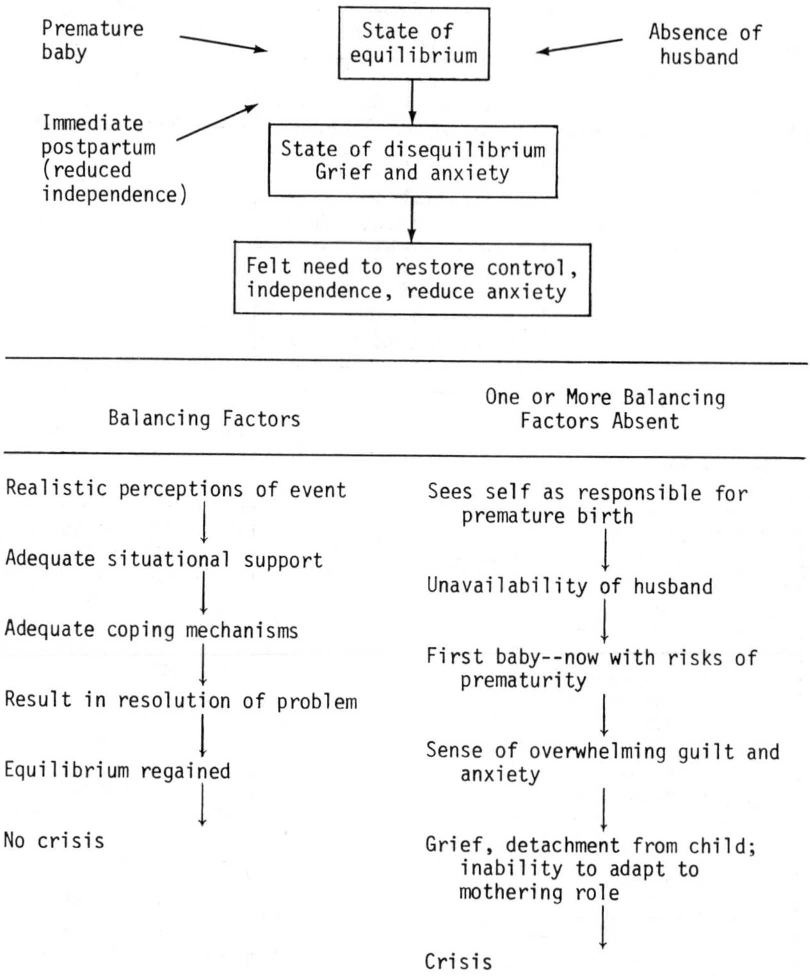

Adapted from: Aguilera, Donna C., and Messick, Janice M., <u>Crisis Intervention</u> (2nd ed.), St. Louis, 1974, the C. V. Mosby Co.

Figure 7.3 Case study: Birth of a premature infant. (Used with permission. Adapted from Aguilera, Donna C., & Messick, Janice M. *Crisis Intervention,* 4th ed. St. Louis, The C. V. Mosby Co., 1982.)

hospital stay, she must resume her relationship with it in preparation for the infant's homecoming.

4. She must prepare herself for the job of caring for the baby through an understanding of its special needs and growth patterns (Kaplan & Mason, 1965, p. 124).

When mother and baby are separated at birth, the process of attachment is delayed.The mother does not get to know her baby's unique looks and ways of responding. The process of adapting and adjusting to the "real" baby versus the imaged child is difficult when physical separation has occurred. Consideration must be given to the fact that the mother may have difficulty in the future with the mother–child relationship if the process of attachment is not fostered. Klaus and Farnaroff (1979) have described frequent evidence of severe mothering difficulties with women possessing one of the following factors:

1. The previous loss of a newborn infant, including miscarriage and induced abortion.
2. A fertility problem with no living children.
3. A previous seriously ill newborn infant.
4. Primiparity if younger than 17 or older than 38 years.
5. A medical problem with which the infant may be affected, such as Rh disease, toxemia, or diabetes.
6. The unmarried mother (pp. 4, 8).

Elizabeth's grief process may be exhibited by a variety of somatic symptoms and anxieties as previously described by Lindemann. Many health personnel feel that tranquilizers should not be given to the client during this time as it may impede the normal grieving process. The nurse needs to provide direction to her in terms of the need to allow her feelings to come forth. Adequate rest is important during this time of stress, and nursing care should be planned to promote a quiet, calm environment. Many clients may benefit from a single room in order to allow privacy during the time sorting out of events is occurring. It may be important for Elizabeth to recall in detail the events of her pregnancy, labor, and delivery. Many women need to repeat their experiences in order to validate and confirm the happenings.

Elizabeth and Jack have also been separated quite soon after the baby's delivery in order for Jack to accompany the baby to the regional hospital. During this time of separation, they have lost the close contact with one another for mutual support. Jack will need to be informed by the staff at the regional center as to the infant's condition. As much opportunity as possible should be provided for Jack to see and touch the baby. Jack needs a clear explanation of the baby's health problem, usual treatment approach, and nursing care that the baby will receive. Visiting policies should be described and a telephone number provided so that Jack and Elizabeth will have access to information and contact with their baby as frequently as possible. Jack may be somewhat overwhelmed as he is trying to take in all of the information about the baby to take to Elizabeth. The burden of parenthood in this situation may have found Jack totally unprepared. The staff needs to assess Jack's reaction to the premature birth of his son and provide him with needed support.

Elizabeth needs to be assured that contact will be kept with the regional center to provide her with continuous information concerning her baby. Some centers have experimented with videotaping the baby in the special care nursery and sending the tape to the family in the outlying area (Perez, 1981). This attempt to provide greater contact with the mother and infant through visual aids can also be accomplished by allowing a family member or staff person to photograph the baby in the unit. The process of attachment will be enhanced by whatever means of interaction with the infant that can be realistically provided. Since Elizabeth had been planning to breast-feed her baby, she can be encouraged to pump her breasts and bring in or send frozen breast milk to the unit. As the infant's condition improves, he will benefit from the constituents provided in the breast milk. Elizabeth may then feel a greater sense of involvement with her child if she is encouraged to participate in his care through providing feedings. The nurse caring for Elizabeth needs to recognize that many women who are separated from their infants feel a detachment from them (Stone, 1971). Elizabeth should be made aware that this is normal and can be dealt with. Rejection of the high-risk child is often a response to a complexity of factors: the woman is giving up her dreams of the imagined child and must cope with the reality of the baby and his needs; she may be dealing with guilt and anger at this unexpected event; and the family may be experiencing difficulty in trying to attach to an infant that may not live—it is natural to protect yourself from being hurt. By not acknowledging the infant and relating to it, many families may feel that the loss of the infant will be less acute. It is also important to recognize that past experiences and coping patterns will have an impact on the present situation and the way it is handled.

In considering Elizabeth's stresses, it might be helpful to resort to Caplan's framework, previously cited. Nursing intervention can promote equilibrium through providing emotional support, clear information, and provision for opportunities for maternal–infant attachment.

Death of the Infant

The death of an infant brings forth another crisis state, with parents reacting intensely. Often the early reactions are shock, disbelief, and denial. Each individual, however, may respond in a unique fashion depending on former unresolved guilt and/or grieving. Occasionally a parent cannot grasp the death and will respond initially with anger and hostility. The nurse may be the likely one that the parent vents his or her anger towards with remarks such as: "What can you do to help me?" or "You didn't tell me my baby was going to die." Feelings of guilt are also common. The previous attitude held toward the unborn child if ambivalent or negative may cause particularly strong guilt reactions following the infant's death. It is essential for the nurse to investigate what response the parent is experiencing and maintain an accepting attitude. It is critical for the nurse to realize that the death of a child has effects beyond the parents to other family members and friends and has an impact on family life plans. Dr. George A. Little (Slade, 1980, p. 11), Chairman of Dartmouth Medical School's Department of Maternal and Child Health has pointed out that "Americans are having fewer kids, making each death more poignant. They plan their families, so death destroys their life timetables." With many women beginning or continuing childbearing at a later age, this point becomes particularly significant.

Many health professionals now recognize the importance of parents viewing the infant following death. Klaus and Kennell (1976) believe that some parents need to see proof that the infant actually died. Prior to birth, the parents have a vision of the healthy, imagined child. Viewing the infant following death will help the parent to recognize the reality of the birth and surrounding events leading to the death. Often the fantasy the parents have concerning the appearance of the infant is worse than the actual characteristics of the infant. The opportunity to see and touch the child may dispel the fear that the parents have produced a "monster." This may have a profound impact on the couple's ability to deal with future pregnancies. Parents need to be reassured that the initial reaction they are experiencing with the infant's death is to be expected. Often parents feel that the response they are having is abnormal and they are in need of intense psychiatric help. The staff caring for the family must examine the impact of the death in relation to the parents' coping mechanisms and provide emotional support and/or referral if appropriate.

The staff caring for the family must carefully examine their own feelings toward infant death. Often parents have reported dealing with staff who avoid the topic of the baby, avoid the parents, or discourage viewing and touching the child. Very often parents experience lack of support and follow-up in the community. Too frequently, the death of the infant is dealt with lightly and with coldness and indifference. The parents are presented with such callous remarks as "you can always have another baby, you're still young," or "you didn't know the child, so you won't miss it." Parents need to feel that the nurse has an appreciation of their feelings. The nurse who can express concern and empathy toward the parents can provide great comfort.

The upheaval in a family following an infant's death is extremely stressful. The crisis may bring to a head underlying tensions that can lead to separation, divorce, or suicide. Siblings often have many concerns and questions following the death. The sibling may assume responsibility in some way for the death. The parents may need assistance in helping other children in the family to understand the death. The children need to be able to ask questions and release their emotions. Parents need to be advised to be honest and not make up stories or fairy tales as an explanation. Children, just like adults, may express their grief in a variety of ways. The individuality of the child needs to be respected as he or she works through the grief process at his or her own unique pace.

It is not uncommon for couples to try to deal with the loss and emptiness by seeking to have another pregnancy closely following the infant's death. Couples need to be advised that it is beneficial for them to work through the loss of the deceased infant before trying to attach to a subsequent unborn child and newborn.

In their state of grief, parents often find their relationships with family and friends strained. The activities of daily living seem meaningless and tedious. Some community support groups have been established in recent years to assist families in coping following the death of a child. One such group, the Compassionate Friends, has become a national organization with several local chapters. Parents participating in the organization have had the common experience of losing a child. The group offers friendship, understanding, and support to the grieving parents.

The nurse caring for the family following infant death can be instrumental in supporting the family and directing them to community groups for follow-up care. The nurse can clarify information for the family and guide them in their recognition of the normality of their response. The importance of facilitating the grief reaction cannot be overemphasized. Upon occasion, the normal grief period is impeded and pathological grief occurs, characterized by behaviors cited by Cullberg (1972). Families need to recognize when they are overwhelmed by the

Table 7.4 Characteristics of Pathological Grief

Prolonged overactivity without a sense of loss
Acquisition of the symptoms belonging to the last illness of the deceased
Psychosomatic reactions such as ulcerative colitis, asthma, or rheumatoid arthritis
Alterations in relation to friends and relatives
Furious hostility directed at specific persons
Repression of hostility leading to a wooden and formal manner
Loss of patterns of social interaction
Activities detrimental to one's own social and economic existence
Agitated depressions

Used with permission. From Sweet, A. Y., in Klaus, M. H., & Farnaroff, A. A., Care of the High-Risk Newborn, 2nd Edition, Philadelphia: W. B. Saunders Co., 1979.

occurrence of infant death and be directed to appropriate help. The nurse can be most effective in assisting parents with referral when needed. Table 7.4 lists characteristics of pathological grief.

Summary

In summary, the nurse plays a vital role in her or his interventions with the family dealing with the crisis of infant death. The outcome of the crisis will be significantly influenced by the degree of support and caring provided to the family by the nurse at this time of stress and disequilibrium.

References

Aguilera, D., & Messick, J. *Crisis intervention theory and methodology* (2nd ed.). Saint Louis: C. V. Mosby, 1974.

Caplan, G. *Principles of preventive psychiatry.* New York: Basic Books, 1964.

Cullberg, J. Mental reactions of women to perinatal death. *Psychosomatic Medicine in Obstetrics and Gynecology.* Third International Congress. Basel: S. Karger, 1972.

Dubowitz, L., Dubowitz, V., & Goldberg, C. Clinical assessment of gestational age in the newborn infant. *Journal of Pediatrics,* 1970, *77*(1), 1–10.

Howell, S. E. Psychiatric aspects of habilitation. *Pediatric Clinics of North America,* 1973, *20,* 203–219.

Kaplan, D. M., & Mason, E. A. Maternal reactions to premature birth viewed as an acute emotional disorder. In H. J. Parad (Ed.), *Crisis intervention.* New York: Family Service Association of America, 1965, pp. 118–128.

Klaus, M., & Farnaroff, A. Appendix E-2. *Care of the high-risk newborn* (2nd ed.). Philadelphia: W. B. Saunders, 1979.

Klaus, M., & Kennell, J. *Maternal–infant bonding.* St. Louis, C. V. Mosby, 1976.

Kübler-Ross, F. *On death and dying.* New York: Macmillan, 1969.

Lindemann, E. Symptomatology and management of acute grief. *American Journal of Psychiatry,* 1944, *101,* 141.

Perez, R. *Parental anxiety and grief in neonatal transport: Care beyond physiological survival.* Paper presented at the meeting of The National Symposium of Perinatal Nursing, Washington, D.C., August 1981.

Rubin, R. Cognitive style in pregnancy. *American Journal of Nursing,* 1970, *70,* 502–508.

Slade, M. Infant death and parental grief: Debunking the old notions. New York: *The New York Times,* Saturday, September 13, 1980, p. 11.

Solnit, A. J., & Stark, M. H. Mourning and the birth of a defective child. *Psychoanalytic Study of the Child,* 1961, *16,* 523–537.

Stone, F. H. Psychological aspects of early mother–infant relationships. *British Medical Journal,* 1971, *23,* 224–226.

8

The Implementation of a Family-centered Maternity Program

Introduction

Family-centered care has been defined as ". . . the delivery of safe, quality health care while recognizing, focusing on, and adapting to both the physical and psychosocial needs of the client/patient, the family, and the newly born. The emphasis is on the provision of maternity/newborn health care which fosters family unity while maintaining physical safety" (Interprofessional Task Force, 1978, p. 3). It is a patient-oriented concept, which allows that the birth of a baby is a major life experience to be shared by the family to the extent desired. It is a normal developmental task during which professional care is directed toward helping all involved to remain in precrisis on the wellness end of the wellness–illness continuum, both biophysically and psychosocially.

A family-centered philosophy is one which promotes the delivery of care in ways which assist families in coping with the childbirth experience within the context of their cultural value systems. Thus, the system of care created must respond to the individual needs of the clients and their families and not be bound by rigid and inflexible rules.

It must be understood that the quality of the care is dependent on neither the facilities nor large sums of money. Family-centered care is a philosophy, a concept, and, primarily, an attitude. Changes in hospital care delivery systems have been made, in great part, by the concerted efforts of women, their families, and concerned health care practitioners. These people have asked for a cooperative relationship between hospitals, health care providers, and clients in order to develop plans of care that will meet the needs of women, their infants, families, and significant others.

Family-centered Care: The Historical Basis

Before the popularization of hospital maternity care in the early twentieth century, women delivered at home, surrounded by family and friends. During the postpartum period, the woman would care for her infant as much as she was able, feed the baby on demand, and maintain contact with her husband and her other children (Wertz & Wertz, 1977, pp. 3–4).

Several events contributed to the disruption of this home-based care in the United States. The setting for birth shifted to the hospital with the development of anesthesia and analgesia, twilight sleep (scopolamine), a decrease in risk for surgical procedures (cesarean section, forceps delivery, episiotomy), and development of the medical specialty of obstetrics. The work of Lister, Pasteur, Semmelweis, and others made hospitals places to go for care instead of last refuges for the dying. The organization of hospital schools of nursing, beginning in 1873 in the United States, made available women trained to give care to those in hospital (Wertz & Wertz, 1977, pp. 132–177).

During the 1930s and 1940s, the postpartum hospital stay was ten days to two weeks during which time most of the infant's care was done by nursery nurses, and women were expected to rest in bed.

The work of Ferdinand Lamaze in France and Grantly Dick-Reed in England began a revolution in the way woman would be cared for during labor and delivery. From the medicated (twilight sleep) labors and deliveries under general anesthesia of the decades before and immediately after World War II came a group of women interested in exploring alternatives. By the mid-1960s, women began to request local anesthesia for birth, rooming in with their babies postpartum, and infant feeding on demand. Consumer pressure grew as more women began to attend classes to prepare them for the labor and birth experience. Since prepared childbirth is predicated on the presence of a support person, labor coach, or monitrice during labor and delivery, and since nurses staffing labor suites in hospitals must care for all patients admitted, women asked to bring their own coaches with them. The model developed in France was that of the prepared labor coach or monitrice. This concept evolved into the husband, father of the child, or companion of the woman's choice who would be prepared to be with her as coach. Interestingly, women throughout history have supported one another during childbirth, sometimes in their formal roles as midwives, and they have cared for one another during the postpartum period.

A pioneer, from a nursing perspective, in the development and promulgation of family-centered maternity nursing is Wiedenbach. Writing in the 1950s, she emphasized the value of care that focuses on the social significance of childbearing and the important role nurses have to play in enhancing the experience. Her book, *Family-centered Maternity Nursing,* published in 1958, demonstrates her forward thinking and commitment to and recognition of the importance of nursing care during the entire childbearing year.

As rooming-in, the presence of a support person of the woman's choosing during labor, and extended visiting for the husband, child's father, or significant other postpartum became commonplace in hospitals in the 1970s, consumer demand turned to encouraging hospitals to relax their policies to allow for more individualized care (e.g., flexible hours for rooming-in), sibling visiting privileges, and options such as early postpartum discharge programs. At the same time, exploration of alternate birth sites, birthing rooms, in-hospital community birthing centers, and home births began.

From a historical perspective then, it is obvious that maternity care in the United States has, in a sense, come full circle. While the majority of births continue to occur in the hospital, the setting has begun to be more homelike. Furnishings of labor and postpartum suites now may look much more like those at home than those of a hospital, children are often permitted to visit their mother and new sibling, and the woman's significant other is often permitted to visit 24 hours a day, to share meals, and to participate in caring for the new baby. Nurses may be assigned to care for mother–baby dyads. Hospitals are making every effort to offer all the advantages of home birth, while at the same time assuring women that they have available the latest in technology.

Family-centered Care: The Philosophical Basis

With the enthusiasm that characterizes the eagerness in this country to embrace new discoveries, we sometimes do not take the time to consider carefully enough some wedding of the old and new. Eager to find alternatives to the pain of childbirth, women gave up the advantages of homebirth and care that was family-centered in order to take advantage of analgesia and anesthesia. The road to regaining control of the birth experience has been tortuous and difficult to negotiate.

In 1960, the International Childbirth Education Association (ICEA) was founded. One of the chief missions is to provide expectant parents with family-centered maternity care (1979, p. 1). This organization has provided a forum for consumers and providers to work together toward common goals.

Family-centered maternity care as defined by ICEA "is a flexible concept of parent-centered individualized maternity care" (Haire & Haire, 1975). This care should permit the woman and the father of the child, or a significant other of the woman's choice, to be together during labor and birth and, if the infant's condition permits, to be with the baby as much as they desire during the postpartum stay. Family-centered care implies a philosophical orientation that values the family, however the woman chooses to define that concept, and respects the needs and desires of each of its members.

During the late 1960s and the 1970s, in a sometimes misguided attempt to meet consumer demands, hospitals often created plans for family-centered care that were just as inflexible as the services they replaced. Somehow the underlying philosophical basis of respect for the individual became lost in a deluge of shoulds, oughts, and musts. Just as providers of care had once assumed that it was best for all women to deliver under general anesthesia, so they assumed that all women would want or need to attend childbirth classes and have 24-hour-a-day rooming-in with their new infants.

As the Haires (1975) put it so eloquently, "family-centered maternity care is not rooming-in or rooming-out, it is individualized patient-centered care, pure and simple."

Family-centered Care: Implementing the Philosophy

In the early 1970s, ICEA offered assistance to hospitals in developing family-centered programs. The plan for implementation of the philosophy of care espoused by childbirth education groups emphasizes use of existing facilities and staff (Haire, 1974). The plan for family-centered care using a central nursery was approved by American Academy of Pediatrics (AAP), helping to foster cooperation between consumers and providers of medical care. The third edition of the *Standards of Child Health Care* of the American Academy of Pediatrics (1977) emphasizes the importance of contact between mother and infant and urges policies to support this contact.

Nurses are the primary caregivers in hospitals, so their input into planning for family-centered care is essential. In the most recent edition of the *Standards for Obstetric, Gynecologic, and Neonatal Nursing* of the Nurses Association of the American College of Obstetricians and Gynecologists (1981), emphasis is placed on the nurse's role in providing support for the family, for teaching and counseling, and for developing flexible rooming-in and sibling visitation policies (pp. 27–30). Standards for MCH practice developed by the Division on Maternal-Child Health Nursing Practice of the American Nurses' Association (1973) state, as one underlying premise, that "maternal and child health nursing practice is family-centered."

Many institutions have found it vital to put together an educational program for staff that is both didactic and clinical. Included is an opportunity to address the changing attitudes and values of society as they relate to childbearing and childrearing, as well as current trends in childbirth practice. An examination of how women and families experience childbirth and what their needs are is necessary in planning how to provide for those needs. Information should be included on ways to support families, including those families experiencing less than optimal outcomes. The educational program should also explore how the family-centered program is to function and the role each employee is to perform.

Since hospitals have vastly differing physical facilities, the plan for family-centered care developed by Haire (1974) outlines general requirements and suggestions. Each institution is best suited to determine its ability to adapt facilities, modify the way in which care is planned, delivered, and evaluated, and respond to the needs and desires of the women it serves.

A dialogue must take place for examination and statement of philosophy as it relates to family-centered care. From this, an identification of goals and objectives can take place. Decisions can then be made regarding ways of attaining these goals and objectives.

Traditional maternity units are organized with nurseries and postpartum units operating as separate, isolated departments. Nursing staff is not interchangeable; there is one nurse caring for the woman and another for her baby. It is virtually impossible for this system of care to support a family-centered philosophy. Instead, there must be caregivers knowledgeable and skilled to care for the woman and her infant as a dyad. This is often the most difficult change for staff to adopt. It necessitates an entirely new focus and often a new body of knowledge for those accustomed to working only in one area. The preparation and orientation of nursing personnel to this particular change is the key to the success of the postpartum portion of a family-centered program.

Fathers and/or support persons should not be considered visitors in family-centered maternity units. Nursing personnel must consider the role these people play in the woman's life and include them in the plan of care. This may be reflected in a decision to postpone a teaching program until evening hours, when the father or grandmother is present. Family-centered is just that. It is not merely a change in visiting policy allowing fathers or significant others to be present for breakfast or stay after routine visiting hours. It means truly assessing their role in the family and determining how nursing can assist in maintaining the integrity of the family and support growth.

Family-centered care promotes education of the family, providing parents with information about their infant and support in learning new skills. It allows time for women to explore their feelings and thoughts and to continue the process of changing roles. It is a recognition that women experience many changes after delivery and that these changes require the understanding and support of nurses. It may mean that the woman prefers to sleep the first day after delivery and cannot care for her infant. But the next day she may be ready to have the baby with her all day, eager to observe and learn what this new person is all about. Nurses need to be sensitive to these changes.

More than anything else, a postpartum family-centered program should be flexible. It should permit optimal rooming-in, encouraging maternal–infant contact while recognizing the woman's need for rest and taking-in.

Provisions should be made for sibling visiting, with nursing staff available and knowledgeable to answer questions about parenting and issues regarding adjustments to an enlarged family. Perhaps this visiting can include a meal together in the cafeteria.

If the baby is separated from the woman in an intensive care or isolation nursery, provisions should be made for the woman to feed and hold her infant whenever possible. It is particularly important that contact be established as soon as the woman is able and desires to see her baby.

Early Discharge Programs

For women for whom the birth experience has been an uncomplicated event, an early discharge program brings the advantages of lowering costs, reuniting the woman with older children, family members, and/or significant others as early as possible, and allowing the woman to resume care for herself and assume care for her infant in her home environment as soon as she desires. Community supports are an integral part of the success of such programs and must be available to women to assure safe care for them and their infants (Avery et al., 1982; Hickey, DeRoeck, & Shaw, 1977). Flexibility in modes of care delivery for the woman and her infant postpartum should include accommodation for a variety of length of hospital stay.

Family-centered Care: The Advantages

Fostering the assimilation of a new infant into the family structure, whatever that may be, is one of the chief aims of a plan for maternity care that focuses on the individual needs of infant, mother, and significant others. When a family-centered postpartum program is in place, all women have the opportunity to have their infants with them as much or as little as they wish, so there is no need to isolate the rooming-in client. Since all infants come and go from the nursery to their mothers' rooms, there is no need for two separate nurseries. This also affords women the opportunity for their infants to return to the nursery at night to provide for undisturbed sleep or to have infants with them if they wish. Women can also request as much or as little help as they may need in getting acquainted with and caring for their babies from nursing staff. They also can learn from their roommates, who may be more experienced in child care. Fathers or significant others, too, can participate in care and visit as they wish. Siblings can visit and will feel less isolated from their mothers during the hospital stay (Haire & Haire, 1975).

Staff satisfaction is very important to the kind of care clients receive. Mother–baby assignments offer greater rewards for nurses than the separation of responsibilities, once initial resistance and feelings of incompetence or the threat of change are overcome. Working with infants and their mothers as dyads promotes acquaintance of the new family, gives more opportunities for teaching, and allows nurses to follow through on plans of care. In an institution where primary nursing is in place, mother–baby assignment is most appropriate.

Most of all, family-centered care gives a sense of purpose to care that is oriented toward promotion of the well-being of infants, their mothers, other family members, and significant others. It provides an opportunity for nurses to practice the very best nursing care possible by transcending the routine task-oriented approach.

Summary

There is no one plan for implementation of family-centered care that is applicable to all institutions. The attitudes and needs of the community being served will vary (see Bibliography for resources). It is most useful to establish a multidisciplinary committee to assess these and to plan based on the findings.

The major change that needs to be made in order to implement a family-centered philosophy is attitudinal. Nurses can make a significant contribution to the successful transition from a traditional health care delivery system to one that is family-centered.

References

American Academy of Pediatrics. *Standards of child health care* (3rd ed.). Evanston, Ill.: American Academy of Pediatrics, 1977.

Avery, M. D., Fournier, L. C., Jones, P. L., & Sipovic, C. P. An early postpartum hospital discharge program: Implementation and evaluation. *Journal of Obstetric, Gynecologic, and Neonatal Nursing*, 1982, *11*(4), 233–235.

Division on Maternal-Child Health Nursing Practice. *Standards—maternal-child health nursing practice.* Kansas City, Mo.: American Nurses' Association, 1973.

Haire, D. *Outline of a family-centered postpartum program utilizing a central or regular nursery*. Milwaukee, Wisc.: International Childbirth Education Association, 1974.

Haire, D., & Haire, J. *Implementing family-centered maternity care nursing*. Milwaukee, Wisc.: International Childbirth Education Association, 1975.

Hickey, L. A., DeRoeck, E. F., & Shaw, M. I. Maternity day care program offers economical, family-oriented care. *Hospitals*, 1977, *51*, 85–86, 88.

ICEA. *Position paper on planning comprehensive maternal and newborn services for the childbearing year*. Minneapolis, Minn.: International Childbirth Education Association, 1979.

Interprofessional Task Force on Health Care of Women and Children. *The development of family-centered maternity/newborn care in hospitals*. White Plains, N.Y.: The National Foundation/March of Dimes, 1978.

Standards for Obstetric, Gynecologic, and Neonatal Nursing (2nd ed.). Washington, D.C.: The Nurses Association of the American College of Obstetricians and Gynecologists, 1981.

Wertz, F. W., & Wertz, D. C. *Lying-in—a history of childbirth in America*. New York: Schocken Books, 1977.

Wiedenbach, E. *Family-centered maternity nursing*. New York: G. P. Putnam's Sons, 1958.

Appendixes

Appendix A

The Pregnant Patient's Rights and Responsibilities

The Pregnant Patient's Bill of Rights

American parents are becoming increasingly aware that well-intentioned health professionals do not always have scientific data to support common American obstetrical practices and that many of these practices are carried out primarily because they are part of medical and hospital tradition. In the last forty years many artificial practices have been introduced which have changed childbirth from a physiological event to a very complicated medical procedure in which all kinds of drugs are used and procedures carried out, sometimes unnecessarily, and many of them potentially damaging for the baby and even for the mother. A growing body of research makes it alarmingly clear that every aspect of traditional American hospital care during labor and delivery must now be questioned as to its possible effect on the future well-being of both the obstetric patient and her unborn child.

One in every thirty-five children born in the United States today will eventually be diagnosed as retarded; in seventy-five percent of these cases there is no familial or genetic predisposing factor. One in every ten to seventeen children has been found to have some form of brain dysfunction or learning disability requiring special treatment.

Reprinted with permission from Doris B. Haire, The Pregnant Patient's Bill of Rights. Published by the International Childbirth Education Association, Inc.

Such statistics are not confined to the lower socioeconomic group but cut across all segments of American society.

New concerns are being raised by childbearing women because no one knows what degree of oxygen depletion, head compression, or traction by forceps the unborn or newborn infant can tolerate before that child sustains permanent brain damage or dysfunction. The recent findings regarding the cancer-related drug diethylstilbestrol have alerted the public to the fact that neither the approval of a drug by the U.S. Food and Drug Administration nor the fact that a drug is prescribed by a physician serves as a guarantee that a drug or medication is safe for the mother or her unborn child. In fact, the American Academy of Pediatrics' Committee on Drugs has recently stated that there is no drug, whether prescription or over-the-counter remedy, which has been proven safe for the unborn child.

The Pregnant Patient has the right to participate in decisions involving her well-being and that of her unborn child, unless there is a clearcut medical emergency that prevents her participation. In addition to the rights set forth in the American Hospital Association's "Patient's Bill of Rights" (which has also been adopted by the New York City Department of Health), the Pregnant Patient, because she represents TWO patients rather than one, should be recognized as having the additional rights listed below.

1. *The Pregnant Patient has the right,* prior to the administration of any drug or procedure, to be informed by the health professional caring for her of any potential direct or indirect effects, risks or hazards to herself or her unborn or newborn infant which may result from the use of a drug or procedure prescribed for or administered to her during pregnancy, labor, birth or lactation.
2. *The Pregnant Patient has the right,* prior to the proposed therapy, to be informed, not only of the benefits, risks and hazards of the proposed therapy but also of known alternative therapy, such as available childbirth education classes which could help to prepare the Pregnant Patient physically and mentally to cope with the discomfort or stress of pregnancy and the experience of childbirth, thereby reducing or eliminating her need for drugs and obstetric intervention. She should be offered such information early in her pregnancy in order that she may make a reasoned decision.
3. *The Pregnant Patient has the right,* prior to the administration of any drug, to be informed by the health pro-

fessional who is prescribing or administering the drug to her that any drug which she receives during pregnancy, labor and birth, no matter how or when the drug is taken or administered, may adversely affect her unborn baby, directly or indirectly, and that there is no drug or chemical which has been proven safe for the unborn child.

4. *The Pregnant Patient has the right* if cesarean birth is anticipated, to be informed prior to the administration of any drug, and preferably prior to her hospitalization, that minimizing her and, in turn, her baby's intake of nonessential preoperative medicine will benefit her baby.
5. *The Pregnant Patient has the right,* prior to the administration of a drug or procedure, to be informed of the areas of uncertainty if there is NO properly controlled follow-up research which has established the safety of the drug or procedure with regard to its direct and/or indirect effects on the physiological, mental and neurological development of the child exposed, via the mother, to the drug or procedure during pregnancy, labor, birth or lactation (this would apply to virtually all drugs and the vast majority of obstetric procedures).
6. *The Pregnant Patient has the right,* prior to the administration of any drug, to be informed of the brand name and generic name of the drug in order that she may advise the health professional of any past adverse reaction to the drug.
7. *The Pregnant Patient has the right* to determine for herself, without pressure from her attendant, whether she will accept the risks inherent in the proposed therapy or refuse a drug or procedure.
8. *The Pregnant Patient has the right* to know the name and qualifications of the individual administering a medication or procedure to her during labor or birth.
9. *The Pregnant Patient has the right* to be informed, prior to the administration of any procedure, whether that procedure is being administered to her for her or her baby's benefit (medically indicated) or as an elective procedure (for convenience, teaching purposes or research).
10. *The Pregnant Patient has the right* to be accompanied during the stress of labor and birth by someone she cares for, and to whom she looks for emotional comfort and encouragement.

11. *The Pregnant Patient has the right* after appropriate medical consultation to choose a position for labor and for birth which is least stressful to her baby and to herself.
12. *The Obstetric Patient has the right* to have her baby cared for at her bedside if her baby is normal, and to feed her baby according to her baby's needs rather than according to the hospital regimen.
13. *The Obstetric Patient has the right* to be informed in writing of the name of the person who actually delivered her baby and the professional qualifications of that person. This information should also be on the birth certificate.
14. *The Obstetric Patient has the right* to be informed if there is any known or indicated aspect of her or her baby's care or condition which may cause her or her baby later difficulty or problems.
15. *The Obstetric Patient has the right* to have her and her baby's hospital medical records complete, accurate and legible and to have their records, including Nurses' Notes, retained by the hospital until the child reaches at least the age of majority, or, alternatively, to have the records offered to her before they are destroyed.
16. *The Obstetric Patient*, both during and after her hospital stay, has the right to have access to her complete hospital medical records, including Nurses' Notes, and to receive a copy upon payment of a reasonable fee and without incurring the expense of retaining an attorney.

It is the obstetric patient and her baby, not the health professional, who must sustain any trauma or injury resulting from the use of a drug or obstetric procedure. The observation of the rights listed above will not only permit the obstetric patient to participate in the decisions involving her and her baby's health care, but will help to protect the health professional and the hospital against litigation arising from resentment or misunderstanding on the part of the mother.

The Pregnant Patient's Responsibilities

In addition to understanding her rights the Pregnant Patient should also understand that she too has certain responsibilities. The Pregnant Patient's responsibilities include the following:

1. The Pregnant Patient is responsible for learning about the physical and psychological process of labor, birth and postpartum recovery. The better informed expectant parents are, the better they will be able to participate in decisions concerning the planning of their care.
2. The Pregnant Patient is responsible for learning what comprises good prenatal and intranatal care and for making an effort to obtain the best care possible.
3. Expectant parents are responsible for knowing about those hospital policies and regulations which will affect their birth and postpartum experience.
4. The Pregnant Patient is responsible for arranging for a companion or support person (husband, mother, sister, friend, etc.) who will share in her plans for birth and who will accompany her during her labor and birth experience.
5. The Pregnant Patient is responsible for making her preferences known clearly to the health professionals involved in her case in a courteous and cooperative manner and for making mutually agreed-upon arrangements regarding maternity care alternatives with her physician and hospital in advance of labor.
6. Expectant parents are responsible for listening to their chosen physician or midwife with an open mind, just as they expect him or her to listen openly to them.
7. Once they have agreed to a course of health care, expectant parents are responsible, to the best of their ability, for seeing that the program is carried out in consultation with others with whom they have made the agreement.
8. The Pregnant Patient is responsible for obtaining information in advance regarding the approximate cost of her obstetric and hospital care.
9. The Pregnant Patient who intends to change her physician or hospital is responsible for notifying all concerned, well in advance of the birth if possible, and for informing both of her reasons for changing.
10. In all their interactions with medical and nursing personnel, the expectant parents should behave toward those caring for them with the same respect and consideration they themselves would like.
11. During the mother's hospital stay the mother is respon-

sible for learning about her and her baby's continuing care after discharge from the hospital.

12. After birth, the parents should put into writing constructive comments and feelings of satisfaction and/or dissatisfaction with the care (nursing, medical and personal) they received. Good service to families in the future will be facilitated by those parents who take the time and responsibility to write letters expressing their feelings about the maternity care they received.

All the previous statements assume a normal birth and postpartum experience. Expectant parents should realize that, if complications develop in their cases, there will be an increased need to trust the expertise of the physician and hospital staff they have chosen. However, if problems occur, the childbearing woman still retains her responsibility for making informed decisions about her care or treatment and that of her baby. If she is incapable of assuming that responsibility because of her physical condition, her previously authorized companion or support person should assume responsibility for making informed decisions on her behalf.

Appendix B

Assessment Guide for the Puerperium Based on Crisis Model

I. *Woman's perceptions* of the events of birth and early puerperium:

II. *Events and potential risks from pregnancy and birth:*

   A. Marital status

   B. Gestational period

   C. Age

   D. Gravida/parity

   E. *Threats/loss of reproductive integrity*

      1. Abortions
      2. Stillbirths
      3. Previous pregnancy loss/less than favorable outcome
      4. Infertility
      5. Threats/loss to woman and/or fetus

   F. *Fertility*

      1. Children
         a. Ages and status

   G. *Smoking, ETOH use, coffee, tea consumption*

   H. *Pregnancy events*

      1. Prenatal care
      2. Hematogic factors
         blood type ______ Rh ______ serology ______
      3. Risk factors
         a. Toxemia
         b. Superimposed situational events (diabetes, renal disease, hypertension, etc.)

c. Psychosocial risks (use Holmes & Rahe scale)

I. *Labor and delivery events*
   1. Onset, course, timing
   2. Risk factors to
      a. Infant
      b. Woman

J. *The Infant*
   a. Sex
   b. Weight/length
   c. Apgar scores
   d. Condition
   e. Choice for feeding
   f. Adaptation to extrauterine life

K. *Biophysical tasks*
   1. Stabilization of vital signs
   2. Breasts/establishment or suppression of lactation
   3. Involution of pelvic organs
   4. Healing of perineum
   5. Resumption of elimination
   6. Resumption of normal patterns of nutrition
   7. Restoration of integrity of abdomen and abdominal muscle tone
   8. Resumption of ambulation and self-care
   9. Resumption of sexual expression/control of fertility

L. *Psychosocial tasks*
   1. Attachment behaviors
   2. Role transition
   3. Integration of new family member
   4. Carrying out of special rituals, practices, beliefs, health or self-care measures
   5. Identification of life change events

M. *Resources*
   1. Internal
   2. External

N. *Previous coping mechanisms*

(Appendix B)
Assessment Sheet

Hazardous Event	Precipitating Factor(s)	Date	D/S	Precrisis Crisis Postcrisis	Resources	Change Coping

Appendix C

The Social Readjustment Rating Scale

	Life Event	Mean Value
1.	Death of spouse	100
2.	Divorce	73
3.	Marital separation from mate	65
4.	Detention in jail or other institution	63
5.	Death of a close family member	63
6.	Major personal injury or illness	53
7.	Marriage	50
8.	Being fired at work	47
9.	Marital reconciliation with mate	45
10.	Retirement from work	45
11.	Major change in the health or behavior of a family member	44
12.	Pregnancy	40
13.	Sexual difficulties	39
14.	Gaining a new family member (e.g., through birth, adoption, oldster moving in, etc.)	39
15.	Major business readjustment (e.g., merger, reorganization, bankruptcy, etc.)	39
16.	Major change in financial state (e.g., a lot worse off or a lot better off than usual)	38
17.	Death of a close friend	37
18.	Changing to a different line of work	36

	Life Event	Mean Value
19.	Major change in the number of arguments with spouse (e.g., either a lot more or a lot less than usual regarding childrearing, personal habits, etc.)	35
*20.	Taking out a mortgage or loan for a major purchase (e.g., for a home, business, etc.)	31
21.	Foreclosure on a mortgage or loan	30
22.	Major change in responsibilities at work (e.g., promotion, demotion, lateral transfer)	29
23.	Son or daughter leaving home (e.g., marriage, attending college, etc.)	29
24.	Trouble with in-laws	29
25.	Outstanding personal achievement	28
26.	Wife beginning or ceasing work outside the home	26
27.	Beginning or ceasing formal schooling	26
28.	Major change in living conditions (e.g., building a new home, remodeling, deterioration of home or neighborhood)	25
29.	Revision of personal habits (dress, manners, association, etc.)	24
30.	Troubles with the boss	23
31.	Major change in working hours or conditions	20
32.	Change in residence	20
33.	Changing to a new school	20
34.	Major change in usual type and/or amount of recreation	19
35.	Major change in church activities (e.g., a lot more or a lot less than usual)	19
36.	Major change in social activities (e.g., clubs, dancing, movies, visiting, etc.)	18
*37.	Taking out a mortgage or loan for a lesser purchase (e.g., for a car, TV, freezer, etc.)	17
38.	Major change in sleeping habits (a lot more or a lot less sleep, or change in part of day when asleep)	16
39.	Major change in number of family get-togethers (e.g., a lot more or a lot less than usual)	15
40.	Major change in eating habits (a lot more or a lot less food intake, or very different meal hours or surroundings)	15

Appendix C (Continued)

Life Event	Mean Value
41. Vacation	13
42. Christmas	12
43. Minor violations of the law (e.g., traffic tickets, jay-walking, disturbing the peace, etc.)	11

Note. The higher the score on the Social Readjustment Rating Scale, the greater the risk for a stress response of illness. (See Chapter 1 discussion of the work on stress and pregnancy.)

*Items slightly modified by original authors.

Appendix D

Film Resource List

Adapting to Parenthood. Discussion by parents of common concerns after going home with a new baby. Polymorph.

Amazing Newborn. Portrays remarkable abilities of the newborn. Polymorph.

Appraisal of the Newborn. A newborn assessment. AJN Co.

Babies and Special Considerations. Management of babies with special problems: twins, prematurity, RDS, jaundice. Slides/cassette. Career Aids.

Bathing Your Baby. A demonstration by parents. Helpful hints, comments on observing the baby. Film or video cassette. Fairview.

Bill and Suzi: New Parents. Parents discuss their five-week-old daughter with Dr. Brazelton. EDC.

Birth and Bonding. Attachment between parents and babies. Slides or filmstrip/cassette. Career Aids.

The Brazelton Neonatal Behavioral Assessment Scale Films. Film I: An Introduction. Film II: Variations in Normal Behavior. Film III: Self-Scoring Examination. The Brazelton scale demonstrated by Dr. Brazelton; contrast in infants; last film—use with score sheet. EDC.

Breast Feeding. Anatomy and physiology as well as common problems. Slides/cassette. Career Aids.

Breast Feeding. All aspects of breast feeding. Filmstrip/cassette. Career Aids.

Breast Feeding. The nurse's role in counseling, supporting, and teaching. Filmstrip/cassette. NASCO.

Breastfeeding: Prenatal and Postpartal Preparation. A guide for teaching women prenatally and postpartum. Polymorph.

Careers and Babies. Issues and choices of women. Polymorph.

Characteristics of the Normal Neonate. Normal newborn features. Filmstrip/cassette. NASCO.

Death of a Newborn. Portrayal of parents dealing with loss. Polymorph.

Discussion with Parents of a Malformed Baby. How parents learn about and adapt to a child with special needs. Coping with feelings. Polymorph.

Dubowitz Assessment of Newborn Gestational Age. Dubowitz examination and scoring of several infants. Polymorph.

Emotional Changes and Sexuality in Pregnancy and Postpartum. Physical and emotional changes of parenting. Filmstrip/cassette. Career Aids.

Essential Exercises for the Childbearing Year. Exercises to help the body cope with pregnancy and restoration postpartum. Polymorph.

Family Bonding: Pregnancy, Birth, and the First Hours. Attachment in early hours. Filmstrip or slides/cassette. Career Aids.

Fathers. Feelings about fathering. ASPO.

Gabriel Is Two Days Old. An exam with the child's mother present. EDC.

Having Twins. Basic information on caregiving. Polymorph.

Hi Baby, Let's Get Acquainted. Slide-tape program to help new parents. AJN Co.

I'm a Parent Now. Problems and mixed emotions that face new parents. National Audiovisual Center.

Infant Nutrition. Nutrients needed, deciding what and how to feed, breast or bottle feeding, solids. Film or video cassette. Fairview.

Introducing the Newborn. How babies "behave." Filmstrip or slides/tape. Career Aids.

Learning to Breastfeed. Portrays women in early postpartum hours learning to breastfeed. Polymorph.

Modifications of the Puerperium. Physical changes of the postpartum. Filmstrip/cassette. NASCO.

New Baby Care. Help for the first days at home. Filmstrip or slides/cassette. Career Aids.

Now That You're Postpartum. A film to help women care for themselves after giving birth. Polymorph.

The Nurturing Father. Help prepare expectant fathers for new role. Slides/cassette. Career Aids.

Parent–Infant Interaction: Soothing and Stimulating the Newborn. How to tune in to cues of the infant. Filmstrip or slides/cassette. Career Aids.

Philosophy and Concepts of Newborn Assessment with T. Berry Brazelton, M.D. Dr. Brazelton conducting a detailed exam. EDC.

Physiology of the Newborn. A description of normal phenomena of adaptation of the newborn. Cassette/filmstrip. NASCO.

Postpartum Period: The Mother and the Newborn. Changes and caretaking for the woman. Filmstrip or slides/cassette. Career Aids.

Talking About Breastfeeding. Discussions of common and special problems. Polymorph.

The Ties That Bind. Relationship of parents and infant during and after pregnancy. Polymorph.

When a Baby Dies. How to help families when loss occurs. Slides/cassette. Career Aids.

Woman-Child. Problems and consequences of teenage pregnancy. March of Dimes.

Your Baby's First Days. Close-ups of newborns to illustrate common characteristics as well as basic skills for caregiving. Polymorph.

Your New Baby. For women having a first baby. Filmstrip/cassette. Career Aids.

Appendix E

Film Companies and Distributors

American Cancer Society. Local chapter.

AJN Co. American Journal of Nursing Company, 555 West 57th Street, New York, N.Y. 10019.

ASPO. American Society for Psychoprophylaxis in Obstetrics, 1411 K. Street, NW, Suite 200, Washington, D.C. 20005.

Bullfrog Films, Inc., Box 114, Milford Square, Pa. 18935.

Cambridge Documentary, P.O. Box 385, Cambridge, Mass. 02139.

Career Aids, Inc., 8950 Lurline Avenue, Dept. N, Chatsworth, Calif. 91311.

Department of Audio-Visual Communications, Fairview General Hospital, Room AU1, 18101 Lorain Avenue, Cleveland, Ohio 44111.

EDC Distribution Center, Department 130, 55 Chapel Street, Newton, Mass. 02160.

Feminist Women's Health Center, 1112 S. Crenshaw Boulevard, Los Angeles, Calif. 90019.

The Great Atlantic Radio Conspiracy, 2743 Maryland Avenue, Baltimore, Md. 21218.

Ibis Media, Department HD, Box 308, Pleasantville, N.Y. 10570.

March of Dimes Birth Defects Foundation, Public Health Education, 1275 Mamaroneck Avenue, White Plains, N.Y. 10605.

NASCO Health Care Educational Materials, 901 Janesville Avenue, Fort Atkinson, Wis. 53538.

National Audiovisual Center, Washington, D.C. 20409.

Phoenix Films, Inc., 470 Park Avenue South, New York, N.Y. 10016.

Planned Parenthood. Check local offices for films available.

Polymorph Films, 118 South Street, Boston, Mass. 02111.

Women Make Movies, 257 W. 19th Street, New York, N.Y. 10011.

Bibliography

American Academy of Pediatrics. *Standards of child health care* (3rd ed.). Evanston, Ill.: American Academy of Pediatrics, 1977.

American Nurses' Association, Division on Maternal and Child Health Nursing Practice. *Guidelines for short-term continuing education programs for the nurse clinician in intensive neonatal care and the nurse clinician in intensive maternal-fetal care*. Kansas City, MO.: American Nurses' Association, 1975.

American Nurses' Association, Division on Maternal and Child Health Nursing Practice. *Maternal-child health nursing practice*. Kansas City, Mo.: American Nurses' Association, 1975.

American Nurses' Association, Division on Maternal and Child Health Nursing Practice. *A statement on the scope of maternal and child health nursing practice*. Kansas City, Mo.: American Nurses' Association, 1980.

American Nurses' Association, Division on Maternal and Child Health Nursing Practice. *Standards of Maternal & Child Health Nursing Practice*. Kansas City, Mo.: American Nurses' Association, 1983.

Avant, K. D. Anxiety as a potential factor affecting maternal attachment. *Journal of Obstetric, Gynecologic, and Neonatal Nursing*, 1981, *10*(6), 416–419.

Barnard, M. V. Supportive nursing care for the mother and the newborn who are separated from each other. *The American Journal of Maternal Child Nursing*, 1976, *1*(2), 107–110.

Bennis, W. G., Benne, K. D., Chin, R., & Corey, K. E. (Eds.). *The planning of change* (3rd ed.). New York: Holt, Rinehart and Winston, 1976.

Bishop, B. G. *The maternity cycle: One nurse's reflections*. Philadelphia: F. A. Davis, 1980.

Bishop, J. *Family-centered maternity care: How to achieve it, health care planning for safe, comprehensive maternal/newborn services*. Spokane, Wash.: Cybele Society, 1980.

Britt, S. S. Fertility awareness: Four methods of natural family planning. *Journal of Obstetric, Gynecologic, and Neonatal Nursing*, 1977, *6*(2), 9–18.

Bruce, S. J. Reactions of nurses and mothers to stillborns. *Nursing Outlook*, 1962, *10*.

Christensen, A. Z. Coping with the crises of a premature birth—one couple's story. *American Journal of Maternal Child Nursing*, 1977, *2*(1), 33–35.

Clark, A. L. Recognizing discord between mother and child and changing it to harmony. *American Journal of Maternal Child Nursing*, 1976, March–April, pp. 100–106.

Clark, A. L. *Culture and childbearing*. Philadelphia: F. A. Davis, 1981.

Clark, A. L., & Affonso, D. D. Mother-child relationships. *The American Journal of Maternal Child Nursing*, 1976, *1*(2), 94–99.

Coley, I. L. *Pediatric assessment of self-care activities*. St. Louis: Mosby, 1978.

Dean, P. G., Morgan, P., & Towle, J. M. Making baby's acquaintance: A unique attachment strategy. *American Journal of Maternal Child Nursing*, 1982, *7*(1), 37–41.

Eckes, S. The significance of increased early contact between mother and newborn infant. *Journal of Obstetric, Gynecologic, and Neonatal Nursing*, 1974, *3*(4), 42–44.

Elliott, B. A. Neonatal death: Reflections for parents. *Pediatrics*, 1978, *10*(7), 100–102.

Encounters with grief. *American Journal of Nursing*, 1978, *78*(3), 414–425.

Foley, K. L. Caring for the parents of newborn twins. *American Journal of Maternal Child Nursing*, 1979, *4*(4), 221–226.

Haagenen, C. D. *Diseases of the breast* (2nd ed.). Philadelphia: W. B. Saunders, 1971.

Haire, D. *Outline of a family-centered postpartum program utilizing a central or regular nursery*. Minneapolis: International Childbirth Education Association, 1974.

Haire, D. *What is family-centered maternity care, and what are its goals?* Minneapolis: International Childbirth Education Association, undated.

Hall, J. E., & Weaver, B. R. (Eds.). *Nursing of families in crisis*. Philadelphia: J. B. Lippincott, 1974.

Hall, L. A. Effect of teaching on primiparas' perceptions of their newborn. *Nursing Research*, 1980, *29*(5), 317–321.

Hersey, P., & Blanchard, K. H. *Management of organizational behavior: Utilizing human resources* (2nd ed.). Englewood Cliffs, N.J.: Prentice-Hall, 1982.

ICEA position paper on planning comprehensive maternal and newborn services for the childbearing year. Minneapolis: International Childbirth Education Association, 1979.

Interprofessional Task Force on Health Care of Women and Children. *Family-centered maternity/newborn care in hospitals*. Chicago: American College of Obstetricians and Gynecologists, 1978.

Jenkins, R. L., & Westhus, N. K. The nurse role in parent-infant bonding. *Journal of Obstetric, Gynecologic, and Neonatal Nursing*, 1981, *10*(2), 114–118.

Joint Statement on Maternity Care. NAACOG Statement. Chicago: Nurses' Association of the American College of Obstetricians and Gynecologists, 1971.

Kennell, J. H., & Trause, M. A. Helping parents cope with perinatal death. *Contemporary Ob/Gyn*, 1978, *12*(7), 53–68.

Klaus, M. H., Leger, T., & Trause, M. A. *Maternal attachment and mothering disorders: A round table*. Johnson & Johnson Baby Products Co., 1975.

Leininger, M. *Nursing and anthropology: Two worlds to bend*. New York: John Wiley & Sons, 1970.

Linde, D. B., & Englehardt, K. F. What do parents know about infant development? *Pediatric Nursing*, 1979, January–February, pp. 32–36.

Ludington-Hoe, S. M. Postpartum: Development of maternicity. *American Journal of Nursing*, 1977, *77*(7), 1170–1174.

McKay, S., & Phillips, C. R. *Family-centered maternity care implementation strategies*. Rockville, Md.: Aspen Systems, 1984.

Mercer, R. T. A theoretical framework for studying factors that impact on the maternal role. *Nursing Research*, 1981, *30*(2), 73–77.

Neuman, B. *The Neuman systems model: Application to nursing education and practice*. New York: Appleton-Century-Crofts, 1982.

Newman, M. *Theory development in nursing*. Philadelphia: F. A. Davis, 1979.

Nurses' Association of the American College of Obstetricians and Gynecologists. *Model for utilization of NAACOG standards*. Chicago: NAACOG, 1977.

Nurses' Association of the American College of Obstetricians and Gynecologists. *NAACOG joint statement on maternity care, Supplementary statement (1975)*. Chicago: NAACOG, 1971, 1975.

Nurses' Association of the American College of Obstetricians and Gynecologists. *Obstetric, gynecologic and neonatal nursing functions and standards (1974) including the supplement: Neonatal intensive care (1978)*. Chicago: NAACOG, 1979.

Orem, D. E. *Nursing: Concepts of practice* (2nd ed.). New York: McGraw Hill, 1980.

Phillips, C. R. *Family-centered maternity/newborn care*. A basic text. St. Louis, C. V. Mosby, 1980.

Powell, M. L. *Assessment and management of developmental changes and problems in children*. St. Louis: Mosby, 1981.

Putt, A. M. *General systems theory applied to nursing*. Boston: Little, Brown, 1978.

Riehl, J. P., & Roy, C. *Conceptual models for nursing practice*. New York: Appleton-Century-Crofts, 1974.

Riordan, J., & Countryman, B. A. Basics of breastfeeding. Part I: Infant feeding patterns past and present. *Journal of Obstetric, Gynecologic, and Neonatal Nursing*, 1980, *9*, 207–210.

Riordan, J., & Countryman, B. A. Basics of breastfeeding. Part II: The anatomy and psychophysiology of lactation. *Journal of Obstetric, Gynecologic, and Neonatal Nursing*, 1980, *9*, 210–213.

Riordan, J., & Countryman, B. A. Basics of breastfeeding. Part III: The biological specificity of breast milk. *Journal of Obstetric, Gynecologic, and Neonatal Nursing*, 1980, *9*, 273–277.

Robson, K. S., & Moss, H. A. Patterns and determinants of maternal attachment. *The Journal of Pediatrics*, 1970, *77*(6), 976–985.

Roy, Sr. C. *Introduction to nursing: An adaptation model*. Englewood Cliffs, N.J.: Prentice-Hall, 1976.

Rozdilsky, M. L., & Banet, B. *What Now*?! Seattle, Wash.: What Now?, 1972.

Seitz, P. M., & Warrick, L. H. Perinatal death. *American Journal of Nursing*, 1974, *74*(11), 2028–2033.

Slade, C. I., Reidl, C. J., & Mangurten, H. H. Working with parents of high-risk newborns. *Journal of Obstetric, Gynecologic, and Neonatal Nursing*, 1977, *6*(2), 21–26.

Standards for Obstetric, Gynecologic, and Neonatal Nursing (2nd ed.). Washington, D.C.: Nurses' Association of the American College of Obstetricians and Gynecologists, 1981.

Stevens, B. J. *Nursing theory analysis, application, evaluation*. Boston: Little, Brown, 1979.

Thibodeau, J. A. *Analysis of conceptual models of nursing*. Monterey, Calif.: Wadsworth, 1982.

Trotter, S., & Thoman, E. B. *Social responsiveness of infants*. Johnson & Johnson Baby Products Company, 1978.

Index